DERMATOLOGY

A Quick Reference Guide

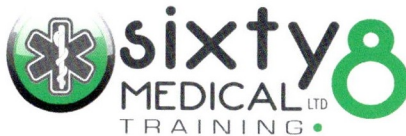

sixty8
MEDICAL LTD
TRAINING •

Fundamentals of Primary Care

Text © Sixty8 Medical 2020

The information presented in this book is accurate and current to the best of the authors' knowledge.

The authors and publisher, however, make no guarantee as to, and assume no responsibility for, the correctness, sufficiency or completeness of such information or recommendation.

Printing history

This edition first published 2020.

The author and publisher welcome feedback from the users of this book. Please contact the publisher:

Class Professional Publishing,
The Exchange, Express Park, Bristol Road, Bridgwater TA6 4RR
Telephone: 01278 427 826
Email: post@class.co.uk
www.classprofessional.co.uk

Class Professional Publishing is an imprint of Class Publishing Ltd

A CIP catalogue record for this book is available from the British Library

Paperback ISBN: 9781859598603; eISBN: 9781859598894

Cover design by Rich Stone
Designed and typeset by Acepub
Artwork provided by JAC Creative Services Ltd
Printed in the UK by Cambrian Printers Ltd

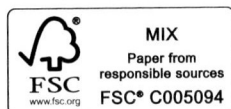

MIX
Paper from
responsible sources
FSC® C005094
FSC
www.fsc.org

Refer to local recycling guidance on disposal of this book.

This book is dedicated to the memory of Vicky Lovelace-Collins. An exceptionally talented and compassionate Senior Paramedic and inspirational role model for her students. Simply loved by everyone she met and greatly missed by her ambulance colleagues, loving family and friends.

Contents

CONTENTS

Acknowledgements

The production of this book and the Professional Learning User Simulation (PLUS) platform would not have been possible without the contributions of some amazingly talented and creative people who share in the Sixty8 Medical vision for quality education.

Main contributing clinical material edited and written by John Kirkby, Paramedic/Emergency Care Practitioner and Sixty8 Medical CEO.

A very special thank you to Lisa Boynett, Senior Emergency Nurse Practitioner and Janice Hiorns RN (retired) for their knowledge and expertise.

Photography: Philippe Sleet. Email: enquiries@phillipesleetphotography.co.uk. Rachel Barrett and Mollana Burke.

Image credits

The following images are the property of Sixty8Medical:

- Page 5 – Anatomy and physiology
- Page 6 – Skin composition
- Page 7 – Epidermis
- Page 10 – Dermal papillae
- Page 11 – Dermis
- Page 11 – Arrector pili muscles
- Page 19 – Epidermal layer
- Page 19 – Melanocyte
- Page 20 – Lagerhans cells
- Page 22 – Meissner's corpuscle
- Page 22 – Pacinian corpuscle
- Page 25 – Glands
- Page 26 – Eccrine glands
- Page 27 – Sebaceous glands (sectional)
- Page 27 – Sebaceous glands (non-sectional)
- Page 63 – Wheal
- Page 69 – Emollient pump and figures
- Page 74 – Eczema cycle
- Page 75 – Emollient pump
- Page 75 – Child covered in emollient
- Page 77 – Common sites of eczema
- Page 80 – Seborrheic dermatitis (face)

ACKNOWLEDGMENTS

- Page 81 – Psoriasis
- Page 129 – Actinic keratoses
- Page 130 – Carbuncle
- Page 131 – Likely eryipelas condition
- Page 133 – Blackheads
- Page 138 – Heat rash
- Page 142 – Chicken pox child
- Page 148 – Mosquito bites
- Page 152 – Tick bite cartoon
- Page 153 – Molluscum contagiosum
- Page 159 – Slapped cheek

We would like to thank the Primary Care Dermatology Society for kindly allowing us to reproduce the following images:

- Page 62 – Fissure
- Page 62 – Macular rash
- Page 62 – Psoriasis
- Page 62 – Nodule
- Page 62 – Petechiae
- Page 63 – Skin plaque
- Page 63 – Pustule rash
- Page 63 – Ulceration (foot)
- Page 63 – Ulceration (leg)
- Page 63 – Vesicle
- Page 63 – Bulla
- Page 79 – Discoid eczema
- Page 87 – Tinea corporis
- Page 87 – Tinea capititis
- Page 87 – Tinea pedis
- Page 88 – Tinea unguium
- Page 90 – Tinea versicolour
- Page 124 – Dermatofibromas
- Page 131 – Likely cellulitis condition
- Page 136 – Hand foot and mouth disease
- Page 139 – Henoch-Schönlein Purpura
- Page 146 – Impetigo
- Page 150 – Lichen planus
- Page 151 – Lyme disease
- Page 154 – Paronychia
- Page 155 – Rosacea
- Page 156 – Scabies
- Page 157 – Scarlet fever (chest)

- Page 157 – Scarlet fever (tongue)
- Page 160 – Urticaria

The images on the following pages have all be created for the book by JAC Design:

- Page 31 – How skin is affected
- Page 43 – Skin healing and wound management
- Page 59 – Describing skin conditions
- Page 65 – Pharmacology
- Page 73 – Eczema and dermatitis
- Page 85 – Fungal infections
- Page 103 – Acne vulgaris
- Page 127 – Common skin conditions

We would like to thank the following for these images:

- Page 1 – Image drawn by S2Synergy Global based on 16th century engraving by Giulio Bonasone
- Page 10 – Blister. By Volty (Own work) [Public domain], via Wikimedia Commons
- Page 10 – Fingerprint © Class Professional Publishing
- Page 14 – Epithelial tissue © Peter Lamb / 123RF
- Page 24 – Granulation tissue. By Linusfox00 via Wikimedia Commons
- Page 27 – Vernix caseosa. By Llapissera (Own work) [CC BY-SA 4.0] via Wikimedia Commons
- Page 28 – Newborn_Milia (Milk_Spots). By Serephine via Wikimedia Commons
- Page 28 – Acne © pimonpim / 123RF
- Page 34 – Staphylococcus (staph). By Matthew J Arduino, Photo credit: Janice Haney Carr, via Wikimedia Commons
- Page 35 – Group A Strep, image property of ©ktsdesign and reproduced with the kind permission of 123RF
- Page 39 – Antibiotic awareness poster © Crown copyright
- Page 47 – Wound healing, image property of © designua and reproduced with the kind permission of 123RF
- Page 62 – Pityriasis rosea. By JoelMills, via Wikimedia Commons
- Page 62 – Papule. By M. Sand, D. Sand, C. Thrandorf, V. Paech, P. Altmeyer, F. G. Bechara [CC BY 2.0], via Wikimedia Commons
- Page 74 – Atopic dermatitis. By G.steph.rocket [CC BY-SA 3.0 (https://creativecommons.org/licenses/by-sa/3.0)]
- Page 80 – Sebhorrheic dermatitis (skin). By Starfoxy, via Wikimedia Commons
- Page 89 – Dermapak instructions, reproduced with the kind permission of Dermapak
- Page 96 – Pityriasis rosea. By Aceofhearts1968 [Public domain], via Wikimedia Commons

- Page 96 – Pityriasis rosea. By JoelMills, via Wikimedia Commons
- Page 112 – Basal cell carcinoma. By Kelly Nelson (Photographer) [Public domain], via Wikimedia Commons
- Page 112 – Squamous cell carcinoma. By Kelly Nelson (Photographer) [Public domain], via Wikimedia Commons
- Page 115 – Superficial spreading melanoma. By Unknown photographer [Public domain], via Wikimedia Commons
- Page 116 – Nodular melanoma. By Hans677 [CC BY-SA 4.0], via Wikimedia Commons
- Page 116 – Lentigo maligna melanoma. By Kilbad, via Wikimedia Commons
- Page 117 – Acral lentiginous melanoma. By Will Blake [CC BY-SA 3.0], via Wikimedia Commons
- Page 117 – Acral lentiginous melanoma (nail). Reproduced with the kind permission of Aim Melanoma.
- Page 124 – Actinic keratoses. By Future FamDoc [CC BY-SA 4.0], via Wikimedia Commons
- Page 124 – Seborrhoeic keratoses. By Lmbuga [Public domain], via Wikimedia Commons

Every effort has been made to secure permission to reproduce copyright images. If any have been inadvertently overlooked, the copyright holders are invited to contact Class Professional Publishing and the omission will be rectified in the next printing as well as all further editions.

Introduction

Rashes and skin conditions are extremely common clinical presentations which can be a minefield for clinicians to diagnose and treat. Some diagnoses can be very clear where as other signs and symptoms form part of an underlying infection or skin reaction.

This resource begins with a concise anatomy and physiology overview starting at the cellular level and leading to the complete detailed structure of skin. Understanding this section is essential to ensure correct diagnosis of dermatological conditions and identification of certain key characteristics and location of rashes to aid relevant treatment plans.

It aims to summarise the useful and common knowledge within a user-friendly format.

We recognise the varied experience and professional confidence of the learner and that there may be restrictions within your own professional registration. Relevant case studies for practice can also be found in the Primary Care PLUS clinic: https://www.sixty8medical.co.uk/the-plus-system/primary-care-plus.

Paediatrics	Respiratory	Dermatology	Wound & MSK
SHAUN TEST (16)	**Tabatha (39)** Shortness of breath	**Margaret (76)** Pustule rash - unwell	**Frank (30)** Knee pain
Alice (5) Ear pain - Right side		**DAVID (56)** Pustule rash - unwell	**Betty (70)** Knee pain
Amelia (15) Feeling unwell		**Marcus (66)** Pustule rash - unwell	**Shaun (19)** Painful Left elbow
Grace (8) Lower abdominal pain		**Evie (29)** Insect bite	**Shaun (24)** Painful Left elbow
Ronnie (2) Cough- generally unwell			
Paediatrics	Respiratory	Dermatology	Wound & MSK
Ear, Nose and Throat	Gastrointestinal	Eyes	Obstetrics
Walk In Clinic (Random)	BLANK TEMPLATE FOLDER		

All of the reference material supplied can also be logged as CPD evidence via your CPD notebook and shown within your professional portfolio (https://www.sixty8medical.co.uk/the-plus-system/primary-care-plus). NMC reflection and CPD log forms are also available to use.

Also included is further reading material, links and supporting information from reputable institutions and common guidelines on best practice. This book is aimed to be a quick reference guide to provide practitioners with an overall understanding of dermatology. Please also refer to the references section in the back of this book for further reading should you wish to expand your knowledge of specific topics.

There may be local variations regarding drugs administration or dosage, general treatments or immunisation protocols, so it is always advisable to confirm your local policies and use this module as a guide rather than an **absolute reference**.

Some useful links are provided here for clarification of drugs.

Useful Link

Management and treatment of common infections guidance for primary care
See Public Health England, 2019. Available at: https://www.gov.uk/government/publications/managing-common-infections-guidance-for-primary-care

Useful Link

Summary tables of infections in primary care
See NICE, 2019a. Available at: https://www.nice.org.uk/about/what-we-do/our-programmes/nice-guidance/antimicrobial-prescribing-guidelines

Useful Link

NICE Clinical Skill Summaries
See, NICE, 2019b. Available at: cks.nice.org.uk/#?char=a

How to Use This Book

This book has been designed to aid readers to quickly access relevant information when required. Please find details of features below. This key should help guide your way through the book.

Symptoms

These boxes contain details of symptoms of conditions to aid in diagnosis.

Treatment

These boxes contain recommended treatments for conditions as well as summaries and information regarding drugs, dosage and specific pharmacology information.

Green boxes

These boxes contain summaries of useful information and suggest actions to consider such as send tests.

Amber boxes

These boxes contain summaries of information which are significant points to remember or consider and may aid good clinical practice.

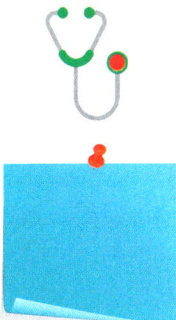

Red boxes

These boxes contain summaries of information which are very important, require action or give immediate instruction.

STETHOSCOPE

This denotes examination. Can be found in combinations of many text formats.

POST IT NOTES

These contain short and concise useful key words, reminders or points to remember.

RED FLAG
immediate
action/warning

AMBER FLAG
warning/
consideration

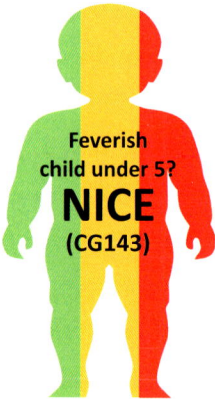

FLAGS

Read and amber flags contain short
and concise key points, considerations
or recommendations.

Feverish
child under 5?
NICE
(CG143)

TRAFFIC LIGHT BABY

Consider referencing unwell children
under 5 years old against NICE
CG143 (NICE, 2019j)

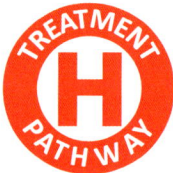

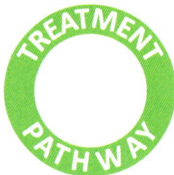

- GREEN
- AMBER
- RED.

TREATMENT
H
PATHWAY

TREATMENT
PATHWAY

TREATMENT PATHWAYS

Depending on the history and
clinical presentations each symbol
denotes the suggested destination,
specific team, speciality or urgency of
treatments:

RED – Direct to hospital immediately

GREEN – Routine referral including
general referrals to speciality clinics.

REQUIRE BOTH PAEDIATRIC REFERRAL & ASSESSMENT IN HOSPITAL

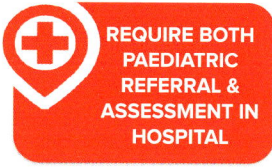

Treatment pathways may have specific emergency instruction.

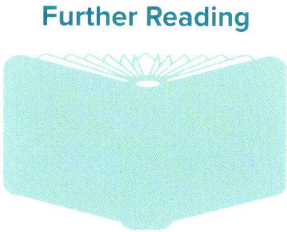

Further Reading

FURTHER READING

These contains citations which link to further reading in the references section and which may be of additional interest.

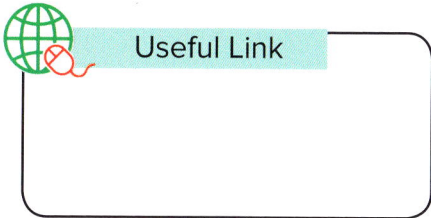

Useful Link

USEFUL LINKS

Contain links to supporting information web sites including referencing material or best practice guidance.

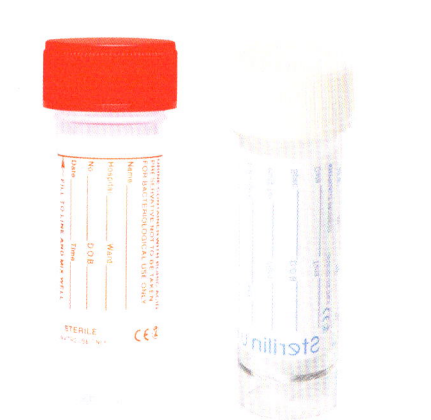

URINALYSIS

Consider testing the urine and sending to the laboratory for analysis. Use appropriate bottle pending age and samples under local guidelines:

- Red top bottle
- White top bottle.

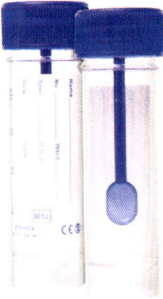

BLUE TOP BOTTLE

Consider sending a laboratory stool sample for analysis of various clinical conditions.

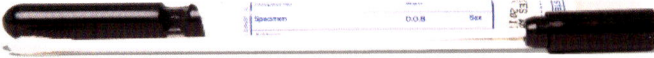

SWAB

Consider sending a laboratory sample for analysis of wounds, pus, fluids, body areas.

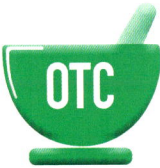

OTC

Consider alternative over-the-counter medications rather than prescription.

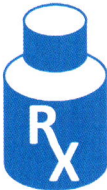

Prescription required.

The Integumentary System

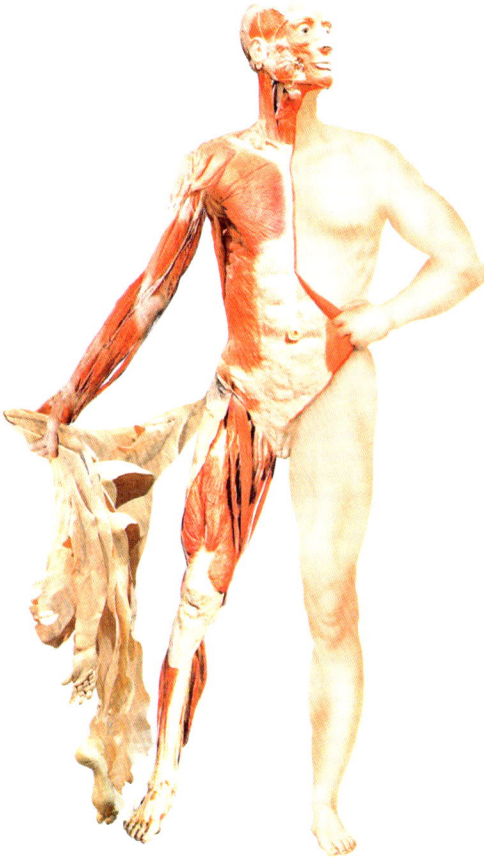

Introducing the integumentary system

The integumentary system is the largest organ system of the body and is continuous within all membranes and linings. Its primary function is to protect the body from a variety of factors which could cause damage as well as to provide essential homeostatic functions.

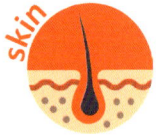

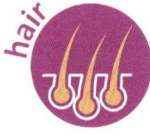

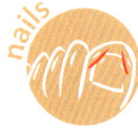

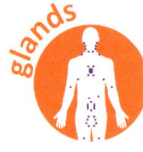

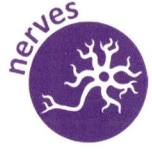

Did you know that ...?

- On average, 14 species of fungi live between your toes
- Sweat is odourless; it's bacteria that causes body odour
- Skin cells are reproduced every 28 days
- Skin accounts for approximately 15% of your total body weight
- The average adult has approximately 21 square feet of skin
- Skin contains more than 11 miles of blood vessels
- A single square inch of skin has about 19 million cells and up to 300 sweat glands
- Skin is thickest on your feet (1.4 mm) and thinnest on your eyelids (0.2 mm)
- Human skin colour is determined by the interaction of melanin, carotene and haemoglobin.

(Forefront Dermatology, 2017; Baidya, 2015)

Main functions of the integumentary system

Protection

- Skin is the body's initial defence against bacteria, viruses and microbes
- Provides protection from harmful ultraviolet radiation and sunburn
- Provides a waterproof layer
- Excretes waste products.

Thermal regulation and sensory input

- Heat – cold
- Environmental stimulation factors.

Endocrine function

- Via glands and hormones.

Vitamin D synthesis

- Using ultraviolet light.

Storage

- Storage of water, fat, glucose and vitamin D.

Healing

- The complex process of cellular restorative response to tissue injury.

Anatomy and Physiology

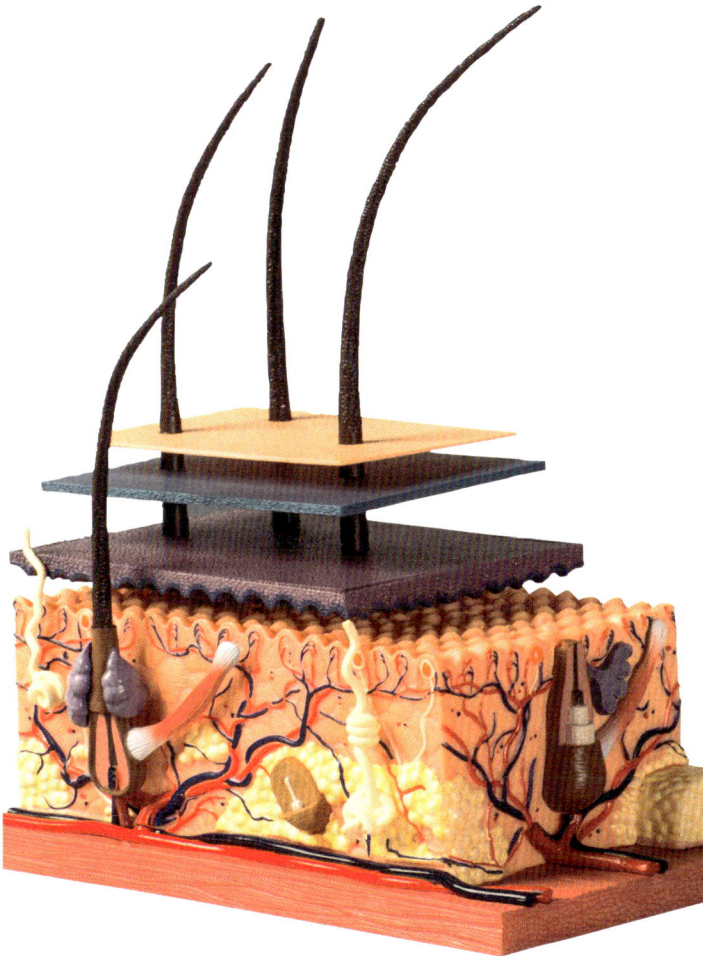

Overview of skin composition

Literature varies when stating how many layers of skin there are in the human body. Some texts count two skin layers, the **epidermis** and **dermis**, then label the **subcutaneous** layer as an independent structure while others group all three of these together.

For the purpose of this book we will be describing the skin structure as having three main layers:

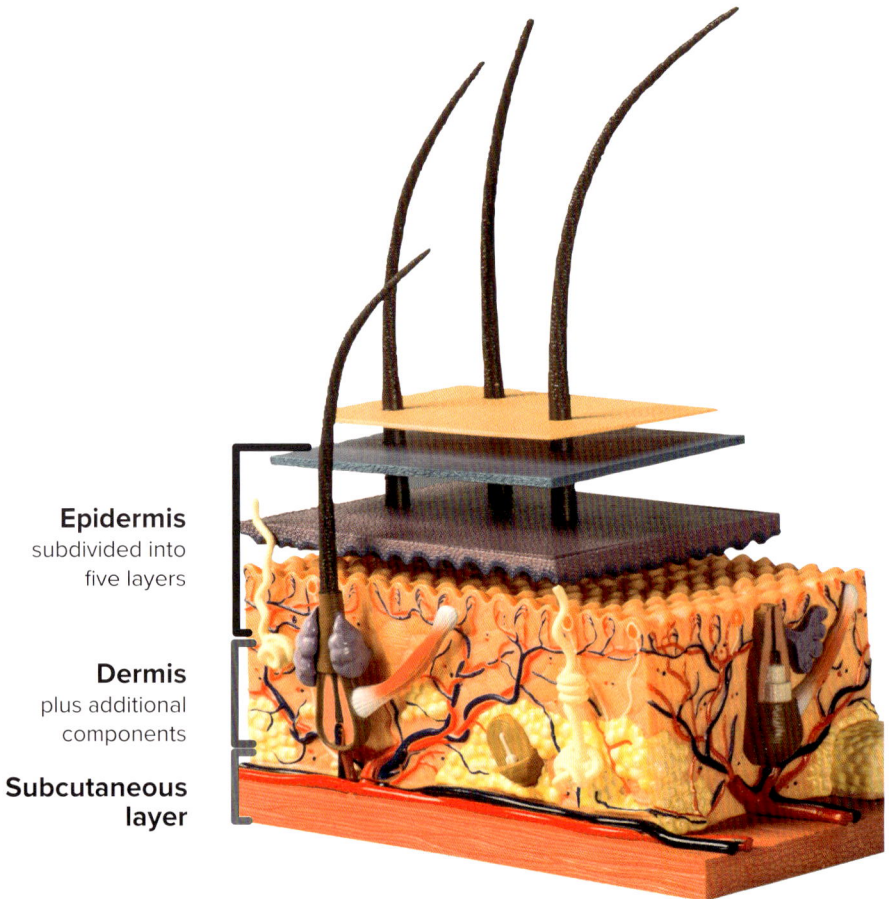

Epidermis
subdivided into
five layers

Dermis
plus additional
components

**Subcutaneous
layer**

The epidermis

The word epidermis is derived from the Greek 'epi' meaning above/outer and is used to describe the outermost layer of the skin. The epidermis is composed of stratified layers of flattened cells which mainly consist of keratinocytes (McGrath, 2016).

Key features of the epidermis include:

- **Stratified** – made up of layers
- **Keratinised** – epithelium in which the cells have lost their nuclei and become filled with filaments of keratin
- **Squamous epithelium** – single layer of flat cells which is often permeable.

The epidermis is constructed of five main layers or strata:

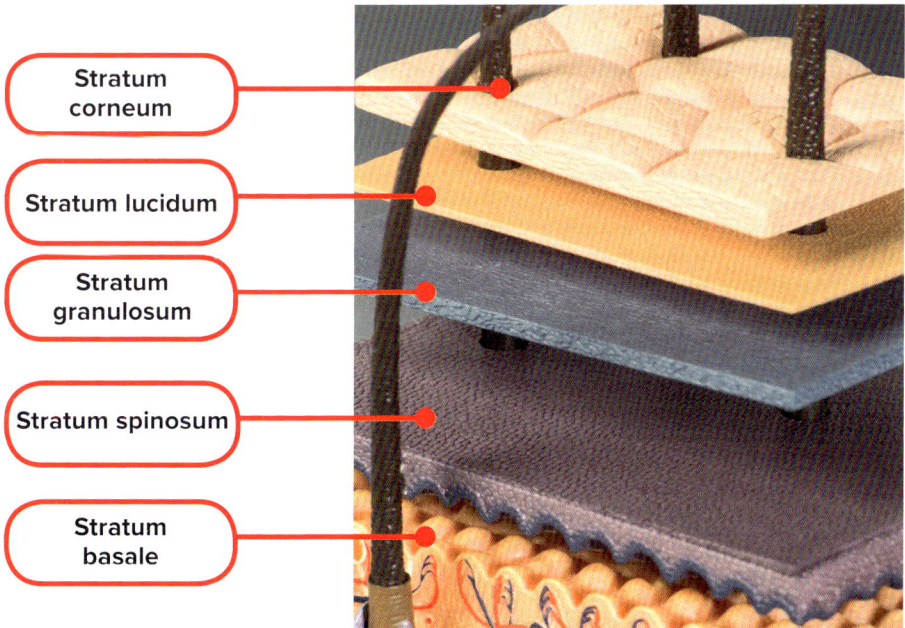

Stratum corneum

Stratum lucidum

Stratum granulosum

Stratum spinosum

Stratum basale

The **stratum corneum** (horny layer) is the outermost layer of the epidermis and is composed of 15–20 layers of dead, flattened cells with no nuclei or cell organelles. The purpose of the stratum corneum is to form a front-line barrier of protection from infection for the underlying tissues and structures.

The **stratum lucidium** (clear layer) is a thin, clear layer of dead skin cells named for its translucent appearance under a microscope. It is composed of three to five layers of dead, flattened keratinocytes.

The stratum granulosum (granular layer) is a thin layer of cells in the epidermis. Keratinocytes migrating from the underlying stratum spinosum become known as granular cells here. As the keratin accumulates, it functions as a waterproof layer of the skin and also forms a thicker layer in order to protect the less dense cells underneath.

The **stratum spinosum** aids in flexibility and enables the epidermis to better withstand the effects of friction and abrasion. The stratum spinosum layer is thicker in areas of the skin such as the soles of the feet and palms of the hands because they experience a greater degree of wear and tear from contact with external surfaces. Langerhans (immune) cells are also most prominent in the stratum spinosum.

The **stratum basale** is the deepest of the five layers of the epidermis and is a continuous layer of cells which are usually only one cell thick. They are layered directly above the dermis and conform to the ridge shape of the dermal papillae. Melanocytes are typically distributed at regular intervals along the stratum basale and their dendritic processes extend to reach keratinocytes throughout the stratum basale and stratum spinosum layers.

The surface cells are flat in shape and dead because they have no nucleus which has been replaced by the protein, keratin. These cells are constantly rubbed away by our everyday activities and replaced by a generation of newer epithelial cells which are emerging from the lower epidermal layers of the stratum spinosum. These new cells are slowly being keratinised as they migrate through the dermal layers to the surface of the skin in a cycle that takes around 28 days for an average middle-aged adult (Skin Authority, 2019).

There are no blood vessels or nerve endings found within the epidermis although its sub-layers contain interstitial fluid which is supplied from the dermal layer. The interstitial fluid provides the epidermis with the necessary oxygenation and nutrients required and its waste products are drained away as lymph.

This process of supply and waste removal is achieved mainly by the shape and construction of the **dermal papillae** which are found at the join between the epidermal and dermal layers.

The epidermis varies in thickness around the body due to the **stratum spinosum** layer:

■ Skin is thickest around the palms of the hands and soles of the feet
■ Skin is thinnest around the eyelids and face.

Further Reading

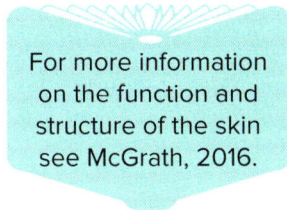

For more information on the function and structure of the skin see McGrath, 2016.

Dermal papillae

The dermal papillae are part of the uppermost layer of the dermis (the **papillary dermis**). The ridges they form increase the surface area between the dermis and epidermis strengthening the connection between them. The main function of the dermal papillae is to support the epidermis but it also greatly increases the exchange of oxygen, nutrients, and waste products between the two layers.

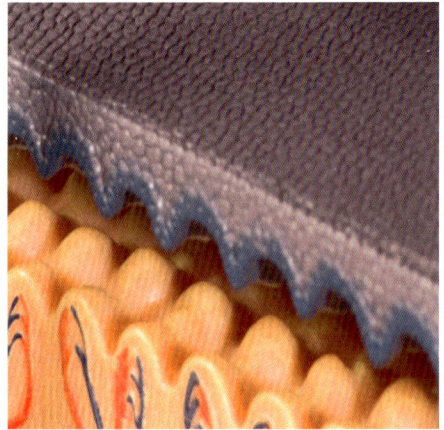

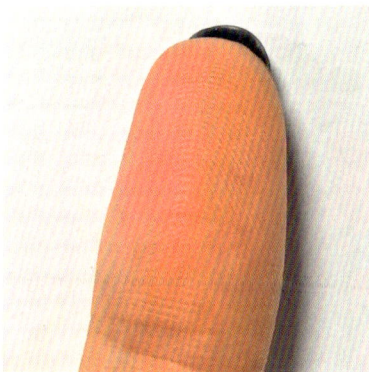

On the surface of the skin in hands and feet the dermal papillae appear as epidermal or papillary ridges. The formed patterns of these ridges are partly genetically determined and start to develop before birth. The patterns remain unchanged throughout our lifetime and therefore determine the unique patterns of **fingerprints**.

If serous fluid or blood has been forced between the dermal papillae and the stratum basale/stratum spinosum via friction or force then **blisters** are formed (Harvard Medical School, 2019).

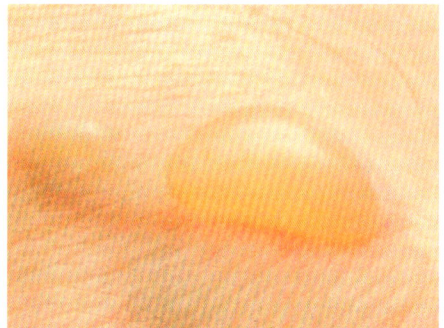

The dermis

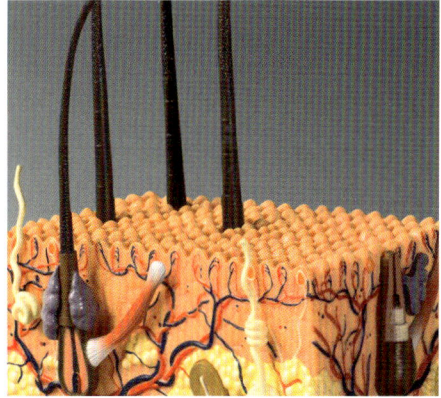

The dermis is a layer of skin between the epidermis and subcutaneous tissues that primarily consists of dense connective tissue which helps cushion the body from stress and strain. The dermis is tightly connected to the epidermis through a basement membrane and its structural components are mainly collagen and elastic fibres. It is divided into two layers (James, 2019).

- The superficial area next to the epidermis is the **papillary region**
- The deeper, thicker area is known as the **reticular dermis**.

It also contains the **mechanoreceptors** that provide the sense of touch and **thermoreceptors** that provide the sense of heat. Blood vessels provide nourishment and waste removal for both the dermal and epidermal cells in conjunction with the interstitial fluid supply to the epidermis layer.

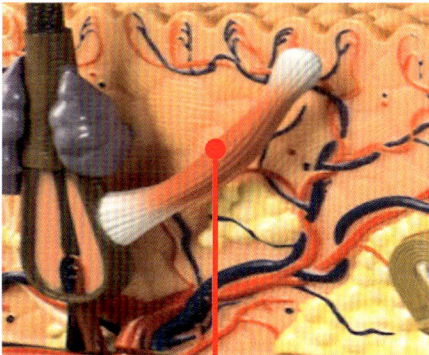

Arrector pili muscles

Other structures found within the dermis are:

- Hair follicles
- Sweat glands
- Sebaceous glands
- Apocrine glands
- Lymphatic vessels
- Arrector pili muscles.

Arrector pili are small muscles attached to hair follicles which contract and cause the hairs to stand on end, causing a 'goose bumps' effect on the skin (Cormack, 2001).

The subcutaneous layer

The subcutaneous tissue is otherwise known as **superficial fascia** or **hypodermis**. The names originate from the Latin *subcutaneous* and the Greek *hypoderm*, both of which mean 'beneath the skin'. This is the deepest of the three dermal layers and is used mainly for fat storage although other types of cells are found within its structure such as:

- **Fibroblasts** (collagen production)
- **Adipose cells** (fat)
- **Macrophages** (white blood cells).

The subcutaneous tissue layer plays a number of important roles within the skin such as:

- Attaching the dermis to the muscles and bones by way of specialised connecting tissue

- Providing support to the blood vessels, lymphatic vessels, nerves and glands that pass through it to reach the dermis

- Padding the body which protects the bones, muscles and organs from physical damage. It stores excess body fat in the subcutaneous layer, which cushions the body and helps prevent injury

- Providing insulation to the body to protect it from overheating or over cooling during changes in environmental temperature. This process of maintaining temperature is known as **thermoregulation.**

(Smith, 2019)

Tissues

Tissues in our bodies are constructed from large quantities of the same types of cell and are classified according to their size, shape and function. There are four main types of tissue, each of which contain variant subtypes. In this reference guide we will concentrate mainly on the epithelial and connective tissue areas relating to skin.

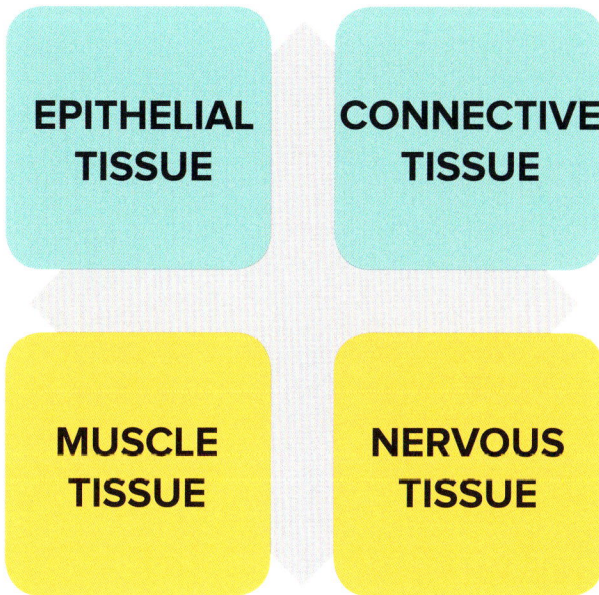

EPITHELIAL TISSUE	**CONNECTIVE TISSUE**
MUSCLE TISSUE	**NERVOUS TISSUE**

Epithelial tissue variants

Epithelial tissue is a generalised term to describe the type of tissue that lines the surfaces and cavities of the body's organs. It has differently sized and shaped cells which can be arranged into a variety of formations and structures. Regardless of the shape, size, or arrangement of the cells, they are still a type or part of epithelial tissue.

Simple squamous epithelium

Simple squamous epithelium is a single layer of flat cells which is very thin and usually permeable allowing small molecules to pass quickly through membranes by the processes of filtration or diffusion.

The thin tissue forms a delicate lining within organs. The cells are flat with a flattened, rounded nucleus. It is also called pavement epithelium due to its resemblance to a tiled floor or pavement (Marieb, 2015).

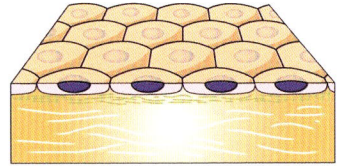

Simple squamous

Simple cuboidal epithelium

Simple cuboidal epithelium is found in organs that are involved in secretion (such as salivary glands and thyroid follicles) as well as those that are specialised for diffusion, such as the kidney tubules. This tissue consists of a single row of cube-shaped cells on the basement membrane (Tortora, 2017).

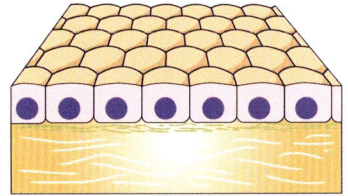

Simple cuboidal

Stratified squamous epithelium

Stratified squamous epithelium is made up of squamous (flattened) epithelial cells arranged in multiple layers upon a basal membrane. Multiple layers adhere to one another maintaining structural integrity, but only the bottom layer connects to the basement membrane (Tortora, 2017). This type of epithelium can either be keratinised or non-keratined.

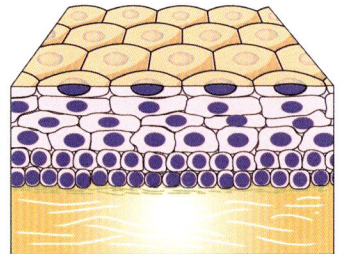

Stratified squamous

Keratinised stratified epithelium

Keratinised stratified epithelium refers to an outer layer of skin cells which have died and become dry. The cells have lost their nuclei but contain **keratin** which helps make this a tough layer and protects the tissues that lie underneath. This contributes to the skin's waterproof property (Pavelka, 2010).

Non-keratinised stratified epithelium

Examples of **non-keratinised stratified squamous epithelium** include:
- Mucosa of the oral cavity, oesophagus and anal cavity
- Foreskin
- Internal portion of the lips.

They must be kept moist by bodily secretions to prevent them from drying out.

Transitional epithelium

This type of tissue is found within the lining of the genitourinary system around the urinary tract and bladder. It consists of multiple layers of stratified epithelium and the cells are able to contract and expand which allows for stretching as the bladder fills (Marieb, 2015).

Connective tissue

Adipose tissue

This is basically fat. It is an anatomical term for loose connective tissue composed of **adipocytes**. It usually contributes to around 20–25% of body weight in adults who have an average body mass index (BMI). Its main role is to store energy in the form of fat although it also cushions and insulates the body.

White adipose tissue is more prevalent in obese people and usually less prevalent in patients who are underweight.

Adipose tissue also releases the hormone **leptin** which advises the brain regarding appetite etc.

Brown adipose tissue is found in new born babies and works differently from white adipose tissue. It has a much better blood supply via the capillaries network and its metabolism generates heat rather than energy.

Areolar tissues

These connective tissues hold organs in place and attach epithelial tissue to other underlying tissues. It also serves as a water and salts reservoir for surrounding tissues.

Almost all cells obtain their nutrients from and release their waste into areolar connective tissue.

Cells and key components

Understanding the anatomy and physiology of the cells and variant components of the integumentary system and their common characteristics offers a mechanical reasoning to relate to what is actually happening within the dermal layers (Marieb, 2015). Age is an important consideration here. The immature physical developmental stage of an infant's skin tells us that they are not as efficient in heat regulation as their parents, so the alarming rash that occurred when the child was in the bath has often disappeared by the time the worried parent presents them to you (Foster, 1969). With older age, the dermal layers, especially the subcutaneous layers, become thinner and are therefore prone to becoming dry and flaky as well as taking longer to heal (Farage, 2013).

The diagnosis of most skin conditions is considered as a descriptive term of the appearance, the history and the location of the rash. A thorough physical examination should focus on the appearance of the rash, the distribution across the body and the symmetry (Onselen, 2016). This should also help ensure any additional complications are quickly identified, and determine if the rash is a primary problem, a secondary reaction to a systemic problem or a normal response as part of a healing process.

Keratinocytes

A **keratinocyte** is the predominant cell type in the epidermis constituting 90% of the cells found there. Keratinocytes found in the basal layer (**stratum basale**) of the skin are sometimes referred to as basal cells or basal keratinocytes (McGrath, 2016).

Keratinocytes are the key structural material for making up the outer layers of human skin.

- Keratinocytes that form in the stratum basale migrate through the epidermis towards the surface in a journey which takes approximately 14 days
- During this process they are filled with a variety of proteins including keratin which protects epithelial cells from damage or stress.

(Ovaere, 2009)

The primary function of keratinocytes is the formation of a barrier against environmental damage by:

- Bacteria
- Parasites
- Heat
- Radiation
- Water loss.

If bacteria start to invade the upper layers of the epidermis, keratinocytes can react and attract leucocytes to the site of pathogen invasion.

Melanocytes

Melanocytes are specialised cells distributed in the skin and other epithelial surfaces. A primary function of melanocytes is to produce a dark substance called **melanin**. Melanin is absorbed by the keratinocytes in the epidermal layers to form a melanin unit that reacts by making the skin darker, which gives protection from the ultraviolet (**UV**) light and radiation from the sun.

In the skin, melanocytes are typically distributed at regular intervals along the basal layer of the epidermis (stratum basale) and their dendritic processes extend to reach many keratinocytes throughout the stratum basale and stratum spinosum (Tsatmali, 2002).

stratum basale

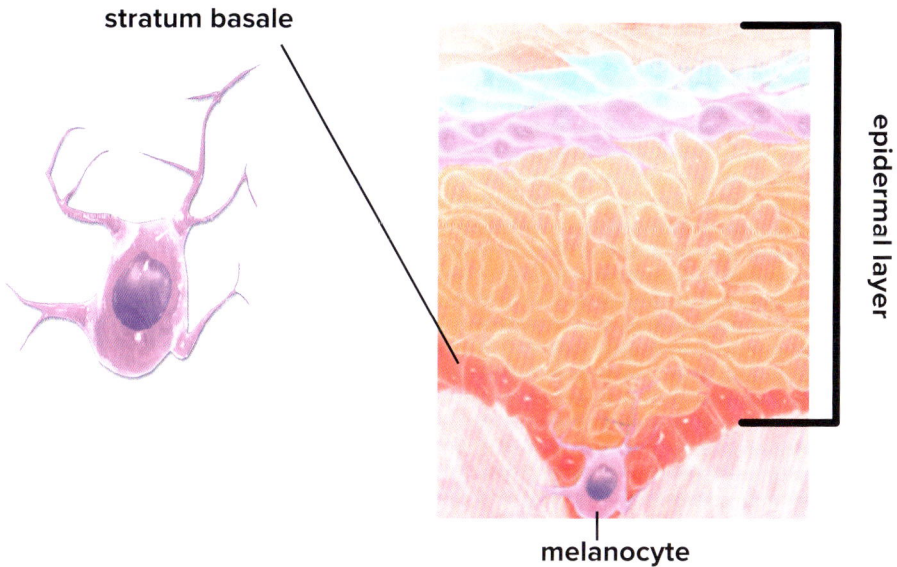

epidermal layer

melanocyte

The number of melanocytes does not determine skin colour. Instead, the number, size and distribution of melanosomes produced by the melanocytes determines skin colour so people with pale skin have fewer melanosomes packaged into the skin whereas people with darker skin have a greater number which are more widely distributed.

Langerhans cells

These are **dendritic antigen-presenting immune cells** of the skin and mucosa. They are present in all layers of the epidermis except the stratum corneum and are most prominent in the stratum spinosum (Young, 2013).

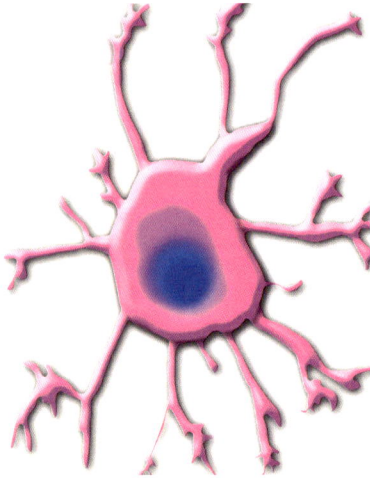

These cells are extremely clever and present an antigen known as professor cells.

- The Langerhans cells are the 'watchers' of the immune system

- They send out immune cells such as T cells and B cells to capture foreign invaders including bacteria and viruses

- They constantly monitor the environment of the skin for unsafe situations and send immune cells to bring back information about any trespassers

- The body can decide to amass a great force of inflammatory cells to fight off the attacker by creating an inflammatory reaction.

Tactile cells

Tactile cells, also called Merkel cells, are specialised skin cells that play a role in the nervous system's ability to perceive pressure. These disc-shaped cells are often found in association with sensory nerve endings especially around the outer dermal layers (Mescher, 2016).

A **Merkel cell carcinoma** is a rare form of cancer that usually appears as firm, painless lesion or nodule especially on the head or neck and frequently on the eyelids and nose. They are typically red, blue, purple or skin-coloured and vary in size.

Neurons receive and transmit messages with other neurons so that information can be sent to and from the brain for communication and action. When you touch an object, the mechanoreceptors in the skin are activated. They start a chain of events by transmitting to the nearest neuron that they have touched something. This neuron then transmits this message to the next neuron until it reaches the brain.

The brain can process the area touched and returns messages via the same pathway to decide if more information about the object is required or if you should move away from it.

The somatasensory system

The **somatosensory system** is a complex network of nerve endings and touch receptors in the skin which is responsible for our sense of touch. It controls all the sensations we feel such as cold, hot, smooth, rough, pressure, tickle, itch, pain, vibrations and more.

Within the somatosensory system, there are four main types of receptors:

- Mechanoreceptors
- Thermoreceptors
- Pain receptors
- Proprioceptors.

Mechanoreceptors

Mechanoreceptors perceive sensations such as pressure, vibrations and texture. The most sensitive mechanoreceptors are **Merkel's disks** and **Meissner's corpuscles**. These types of mechanoreceptors are found in the very top layers of the dermis and epidermis on hairless skin including the palms, lips, tongue, soles of feet, fingertips, eyelids and face.

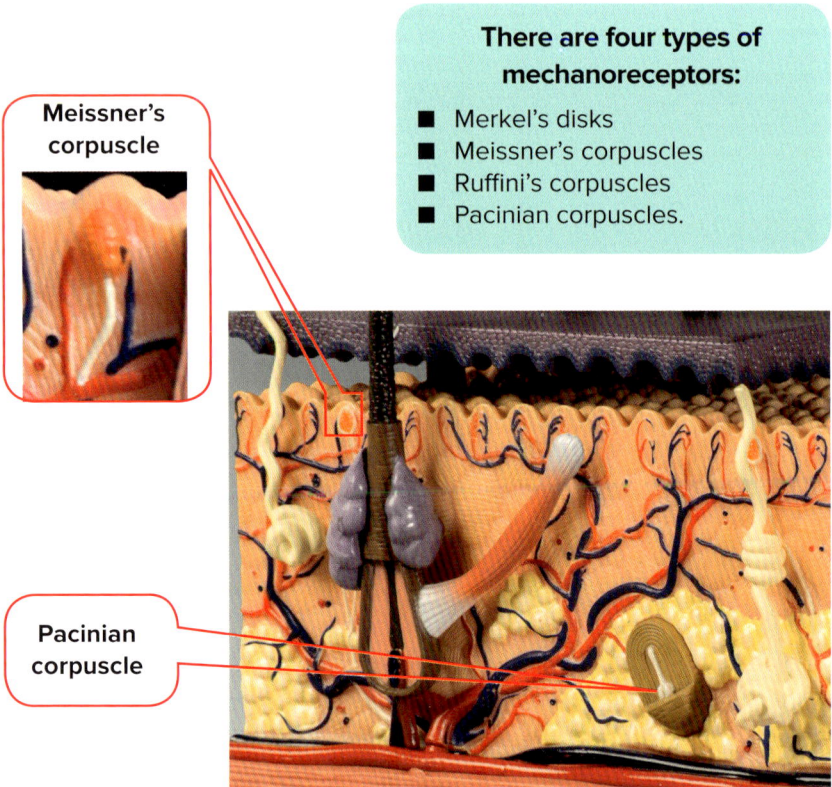

Meissner's corpuscle

There are four types of mechanoreceptors:

- Merkel's disks
- Meissner's corpuscles
- Ruffini's corpuscles
- Pacinian corpuscles.

Pacinian corpuscle

Ruffini's corpuscles and **Pacinian corpuscles** are found deeper in the dermis and along joints, tendons and muscles. They perceive sensations such as vibrations traveling down bones and tendons, rotational movement of limbs and the stretching of skin.

Thermoreceptors

Thermoreceptors perceive sensations related to temperature and are found in the dermis of the skin. As you may have guessed there are two types of thermoreceptor – hot and cold – but they also relate very closely to pain receptors that will take over and stimulate a reactive response to prevent damage being done to the skin and underlying tissues. Thermoreceptors are found all over the body but **cold receptors** are found in greater density than **heat receptors** with the highest concentration of thermoreceptors located in the face and ears.

Pain receptor (nociceptor)

Nociceptors, known as pain receptors, detect pain and stimuli that can cause damage to the skin and other tissues of the body. Their name originates from the Latin word, *Noci*, which means 'injury' or 'hurt'. There are over three million pain receptors throughout the body found in skin, muscles, bones, blood vessels and some organs which detect pain caused by mechanical, thermal or chemical stimuli such as poison from an insect sting (Guinness, 2018).

Pain receptors will cause immediate pain and induce a mechanical response to remove you from the cause, but they also produce a chronic constant dull pain as a warning until the damaged area has healed.

Proprioceptors

Proprioceptors sense the position of the different parts of the body in relation to each other and the surrounding environment. The name stems from the Latin, *Proprius* which means 'own' or 'individual'. Proprioceptors are located in tendons, muscles and joint capsules, which allows them to detect changes in muscle length and muscle tension.

Mast cells

Mast cells are located in many connective tissue structures including the skin where they play an important role to defend tissues from disease. They achieve this by releasing chemical mediators to attract other key components of the immune system to areas of the body where needed. Mast cells are also involved within the process of wound healing so the typical itching felt around a healing wound or scab may be caused by the **histamine** release along with **basophils**, which is an immune (leucocyte) response.

Mast cells have traditionally been viewed as effector cells for allergic reactions that can store and synthesise many mediators when activated by a variety of stimuli (Oskeritzian, 2012).

When mast cells are stimulated or damaged they release histamine and heparin.

- Histamine release from basophils and mast cells causes inflammation in the skin and a greater release of gastric substances into the stomach
- Heparin release prevents coagulation thus enabling blood to flow easily through the inflamed tissue.

Fibroblasts

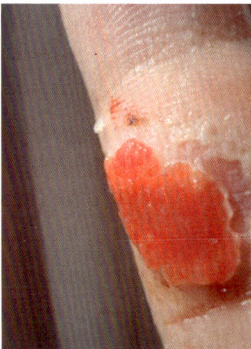

Fibroblasts are relatively large cells found in various connective tissue formations and have several functions but are most prevalent in the healing of wounds.

Fibroblasts manufacture **collagen** and **elastic fibres** which adhere to the open surfaces and are bound together in conjunction with other chemical processes to form **granulation tissue**.

Glands

Glands are groups of epithelial cells that specialise in secretion.

Glands that secrete fluids onto the epithelial surface via a duct are called **exocrine glands**, for example mucous saliva and earwax.

Ductless glands that secrete hormones into the bloodstream and lymph are called **endocrine glands**.

There are three main types of glands found on human skin:

Eccrine glands

Apocrine glands

Sebaceous glands

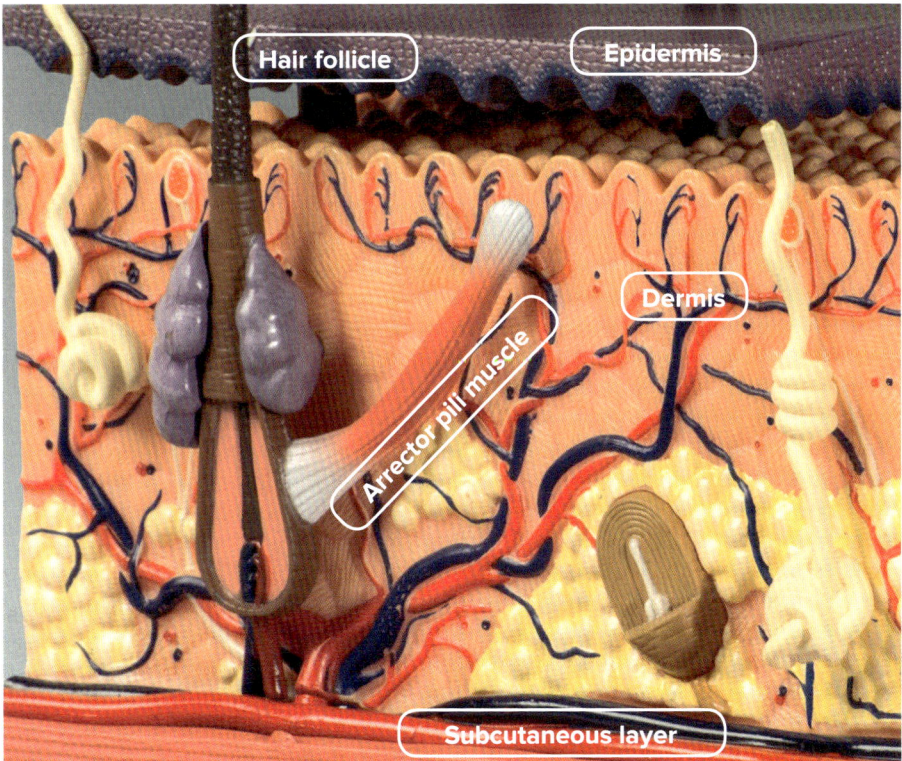

Hair follicle

Epidermis

Arrector pili muscle

Dermis

Subcutaneous layer

Eccrine glands

Eccrine glands are found all over the body but are generally more prolific on the palms of hands, soles of feet, groin and armpits. They are made from epithelial cells and most of their structure sits in a curled formation within the subcutaneous layer. Eccrine glands are very common within the skin and they empty clear fluid onto the skin surface to cool it down (i.e. sweating).

Infants have a reduced skin surface area in relation to body mass which means their eccrine glands are closer together and will function irregularly.

This causes higher temperatures than in adults due to their immaturity and as a result, the infant has a reduced ability to sweat and becomes prone to overheating (Woo, 2019).

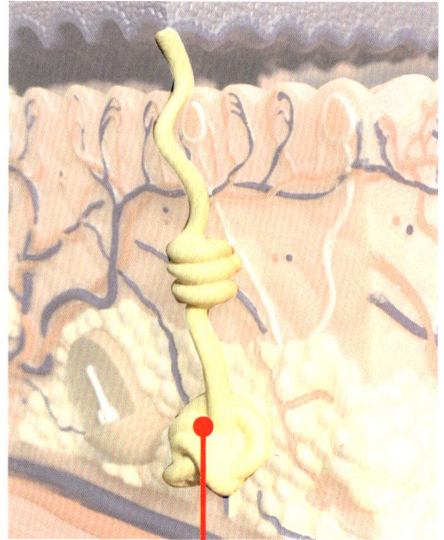

Eccrine glands

Infants overheating may be evident in the form of miliaria, heat rash or prickly heat rashes (see page 138).

Apocrine glands

Apocrine glands are activated during puberty and open into hair follicles. The decomposition of these glands' secretions cause an increase of body odour in adolescents (Mosby, 2016).

The **ceruminous gland** is also an apocrine gland which is located in the ear to produce earwax.

Sebaceous (oil) glands

Sebaceous (oil) glands are made from secretory epithelial cells and are present in all areas of the skin other than the palms of the hands and the soles of the feet where the skin is much thicker.

They are most abundant around the scalp, face, armpits and groin areas where they attach to hair follicles. Sebaceous glands are also found in eyelids, lips, nipples and genital surfaces where they secrete directly onto the skin surface rather than through hair follicles (James, 2019).

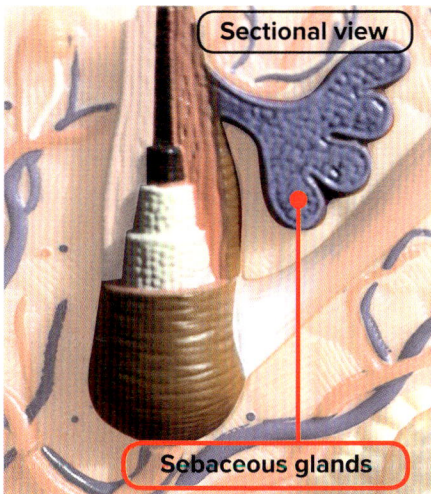

Sectional view

Sebaceous glands

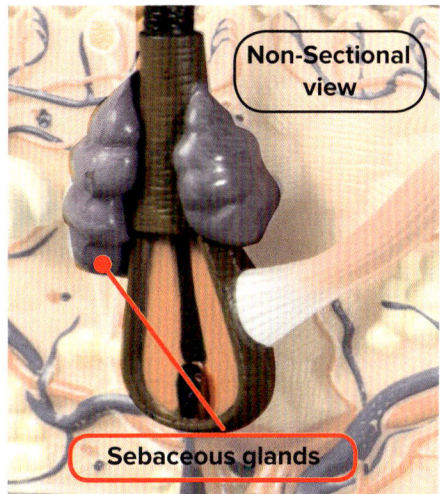

Non-Sectional view

Sebaceous glands

Sebaceous glands become active during fetal life due to the high level of maternal androgens (hormones) and this is most evident at birth where the baby has a greasy covering over the skin called the **vernix caseosa**. This covering consists of sebum and shed skin cells and helps initially to prepare and protect the baby's skin. It is generally washed off at birth or peels off naturally within the first few days of life (Irmak, 2004).

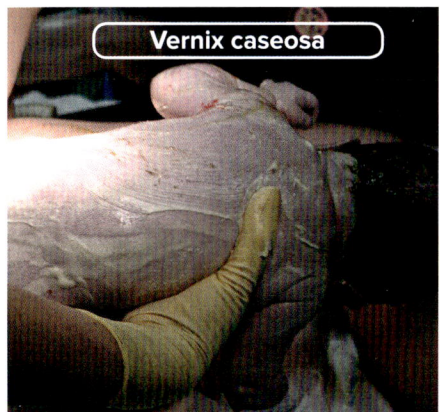

Vernix caseosa

As the child grows the sebaceous glands can become blocked which causes milia, or milk spots.

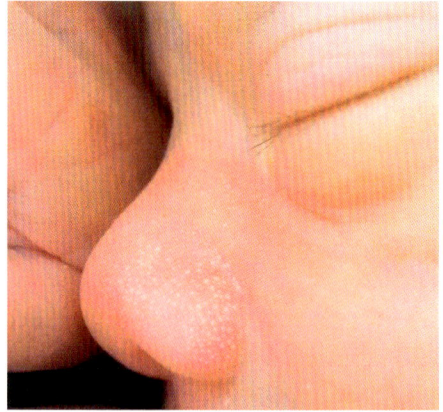

Sebaceous glands and sebum

Sebum is an oily substance secreted by the sebaceous glands into hair and onto skin. It is a multi-purpose substance that:

- Provides a level of antimicrobial protection
- Lays on the skin surface and contributes to the waterproof properties of skin
- Maintains moisture and prevents skin from drying or cracking
- When attached and secreted into hair, the sebum helps keep the hair pliable and assists with cleansing
- When NOT attached to hair follicles sebum provides lubrication on the eyelids, lips, nipples and genital surfaces.

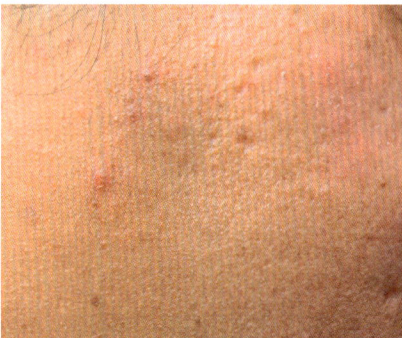

The hormones that cause body changes at puberty also cause the sebaceous glands to produce more oil. If this oil mixes with dead skin cells and blocks a pore, it can produce spots.

Sebaceous, epidermoid and pilar cysts

■ Sebaceous cysts are relatively rare, they contain sebum and originate from sebaceous glands

■ The scalp, ears, back, face and upper limbs are the most common sites though they may occur elsewhere on the body

■ They do not present on the palms of the hands or soles of the feet

■ They are more common in hairy areas

■ They are smooth to the touch, vary in size and are generally round in shape.

Differential diagnosis

■ **Epidermoid** cysts originate in the **epidermis**

■ **Pilar cysts** originate from **hair follicles.**

Both contain keratin but they do not originate from the sebaceous glands.

(Newson, 2015)

Seborrhoeic dermatitis

This a common dermal disorder associated with excessive sebum production that causes greasy, yellow or red scaling on hairy areas of the body including the scalp, genitals, creases on the arms, legs and breasts. It isn't contagious but can be uncomfortable and patients may feel embarrassed or even depressed by the appearance of the condition.

Dandruff is a mild form of seborrhoeic dermatitis and so is cradle cap in infants. This is often treated with specific shampoos or products which contain **salicylic acid** (Eske, 2019).

How Skin is Affected

by Infection, Ageing and Ethnicity

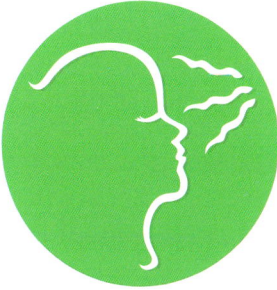

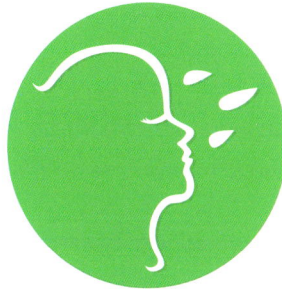

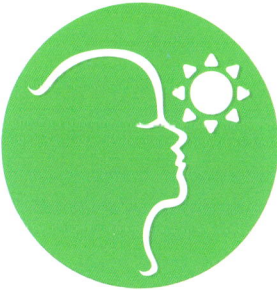

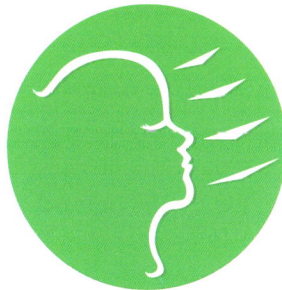

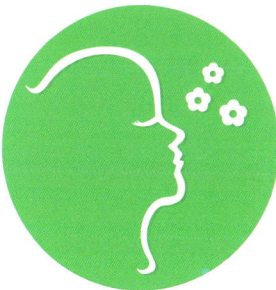

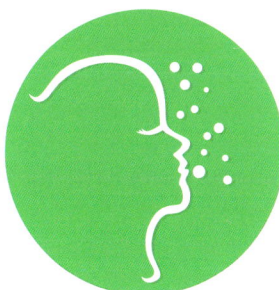

Infection

Bacteria

Bacteria are microscopic, single-celled micro-organisms that inhabit many different types of environments. Some types may live in extreme cold or hot environments. Other types live in the intestines and help us to digest food. Most bacteria are harmless to people and serve a useful purpose, but there are some exceptions.

Both skin and hair are covered in various types of bacteria. Bacteria can form different relationships with the host:

■ **Commensalistic** – beneficial to the bacteria but harms or does not help the host

■ **Mutualistic** – beneficial to both the bacteria and the host.

Some skin bacteria will even protect against pathogenic bacteria by:

■ Secreting substances that prevent harmful microbes from invading

■ Stimulating the immune system into action.

While most strains of bacteria on the skin are harmless, they can cause mild infections such as boils, abscesses and cellulitis while others can create more serious clinical complications such as sepsis or meningitis. Skin bacteria are characterised by the type of skin environment in which they thrive.

There are three main types of skin environments that are populated predominantly by three species of bacteria (Grice, 2009):

■ **Propionibacterium** is found in sebaceous or oily areas such as the head, neck and trunk

■ **Corynebacterium** populates moist areas such as the creases of elbows and between the toes

■ **Staphylococcus** is found on broad skin surfaces and the nasal cavity.

Inappropriate use of antibiotics can create strains of bacteria that are resistant to treatment

Infections caused by bacteria include:
- Strep throat
- Tuberculosis
- Urinary tract infections
- Skin infections.

Viruses

Viruses are even smaller than bacteria. They rely on living hosts such as humans, plants or animals to thrive and reproduce otherwise they can't survive. When a virus enters the body it invades cells, takes over the blueprint deoxyribonucleic acid (**DNA**) and reprograms it to reproduce the virus in vast quantities of ribonucleic acid (**RNA**).

Diseases caused by viruses include:
- Chickenpox
- Common colds.

It can sometimes be difficult to know whether bacteria or a virus is causing the infection. Both types of microbes can be responsible for a number of different ailments such as pneumonia, meningitis and diarrhoea.

Further Reading

For more information on bacterial and viral infections see WebMD, 2018; MedlinePlus 2018; Steckelberg, 2017.

Remember! Pyrexia is one of the earliest signs of a system response to an inflammatory or infective condition.

Staphylococcal infections

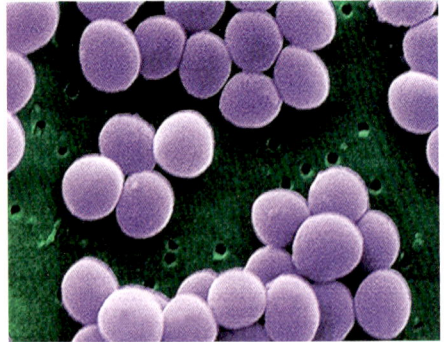

Staphylococcus (staph) species of bacteria are very common. About 1 in 3 people carry the bacteria harmlessly on their skin, usually inside their nose and on the surface of their armpits and buttocks (HPA, 2008). The bacteria can cause problems if they enter the body through a break in the skin.

> There are many types of staphylococci, but most infections are caused by staphylococcus aureus.

Staphylococcus aureus is a common type of bacterium that may be found in areas such as the respiratory tract. While some staph strains are harmless, others such as **methicillin resistant staphylococcus aureus** (MRSA) is resistant to certain antibiotics that are commonly used to treat staph infections. Staphylococcus aureus is easily spread through physical contact but it must penetrate the skin surface in order to cause an infection (Stanway, 2015).

This bacteria is able to adhere to many surfaces including medical equipment which, if entering the body, will cause very serious infections.

Staphylococcus epidermidis is a type of bacterium which commonly causes infections associated with implanted medical devices such as catheters and has become one of the leading causes of hospital-acquired infections which are increasingly resistant to antibiotics (Levinson, 2018).

> **PVL-Staphylococcus aureus** produces a toxin called Panton-Valentine leucocidin (PVL), which kills erythrocytes and leucocytes and can also cause recurrent skin infections, such as boils and abscesses.

Streptococcal infections

Streptococcal infections are any type of infection caused by the streptococcus (strep) group of bacteria.

Streptococcus pyogenes (group A strep) is commonly found on the skin and is not harmful in most cases, however, it can cause infection with immunosuppressed patients. This strain is responsible for a number of diseases that range from mild infections to life-threatening illnesses (MedicineNet, 2019). Some of these diseases include:

- Strep throat
- Scarlet fever
- Impetigo
- Necrotising fasciitis
- Toxic shock syndrome
- Septicaemia.

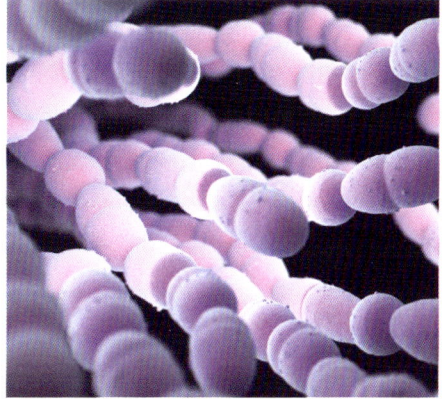

Group A strep bacteria are known as flesh-eating bacteria because they can destroy infected tissue causing necrotising fasciitis.

Further Reading

For more information on staphylococcal infections see Mayo Clinic, 2019a and NHS, 2018a.

Further Reading

For more information on streptococcal infections see NHS Direct Wales, 2019.

Most streptococcal infections can be treated with antibiotics and can be divided into two key groups:

Alpha-haemolytic – made up of two groups, including Streptococcus pneumoniae

Beta-haemolytic – made up of several groups, including Group A and Group B.

Streptococcal A and B

Group A strep bacteria are commonly found on the surface of the skin and inside the throat. They frequently cause infection in adults and children and can be spread through droplets of coughs and sneezes of an infected person, or by direct contact with an infected person or object.

Common Strep A infections are:

- Tonsillitis
- Impetigo
- Cellulitis
- Sinusitis
- Otitis media.

Group B strep bacteria are often harmless and can usually be found inside the digestive system and vagina. They may cause urinary tract infections, skin, bone or blood infections and pneumonia, particularly in susceptible people including elderly, immunocompromised or diabetic patients and pregnant women.

Pseudomonas

Pseudomonas infections are caused by bacteria from the genus *Pseudomonas*. They can be found in moist environments and are mainly found in soil and water. The most common species that causes infection is **Pseudomonas aeruginosa** but only a few of the many species actually cause disease in humans. Like many other bacterial strains these also have a growing resistance to antibiotics.

Pseudomonas infections are commonly found in people who regularly use hot tubs or swimming pools which have not been filtered or cleaned adequately, which leads to ear infections (otitis externa) (CDC, 2016a).

Gram-positive and Gram-negative bacteria

The Gram stain was developed by the Danish scientist and physician Hans Christian Joachim Gram in 1884 and is a staining technique used to distinguish and classify bacterial species into two main groups: Gram-positive and Gram-negative.

Gram staining

Stains and dyes are used to highlight the chemical and physical structure of the cell walls by detecting **peptidoglycan**, which is present in the cell wall of Gram-positive bacteria. Gram-negative cells also contain a very small layer of peptidoglycan but this is dissolved when alcohol is added.

The procedure is based on the ability of microorganisms to retain the colour of the primary stain (purple) used during the gram stain procedure. Gram-negative bacteria are de-colourised by the alcohol causing them to lose the colour of the primary stain. Gram-positive bacteria are not decolourised by alcohol and will remain purple in colour.

A counterstain is added after washing that will stain these Gram-negative bacteria pink. Both Gram-positive bacteria and Gram-negative bacteria pick up the counterstain although the pink colour is not visible on Gram-positive bacteria because of the existing purple colour stain being much darker.

It's worth noting that not all bacteria can be definitively classified by the Gram staining method, so these form alternative groups known as Gram-variable and Gram-indeterminate groups.

Gram-positive bacteria

Gram-positive bacteria such as staphylococcus and streptococcus are found mainly on the skin, upper respiratory tract and oropharynx.

These are easier to kill as their thick peptidoglycan layer absorbs antibiotics and cleaning products more easily, even those that prove toxic to its internal mechanisms. This also makes them easier to destroy with certain detergents. Gram-positive are, however, more resilient between routine cleaning and readily multiply on dry surfaces. Gram-negative bacteria cannot survive as long as Gram-positive bacteria on dry surfaces (Mitchell, 2015).

Gram-negative bacteria

Gram-negative bacteria, such as E. coli and other coliforms and Bacteroides species, are found in the bowel. They have a much thinner peptidoglycan layer and do not easily absorb antibiotics or cleaning materials thus making them much harder to destroy.

Their ability to resist traditional antibiotics makes them more dangerous in hospitals as patients will have weaker immunity and the Gram-negative bacteria's natural defences keep these medications out. Some bacteria even acquire resistance to antibiotics that would normally make it through to their inner cell structure.

Although Gram-positive bacteria can cause multiple problems, Gram-negative bacteria have been developing dangerous resistance and are therefore classified as a more serious threat. For this reason, the need for methods that kill bacteria, both Gram-positive and Gram-negative, is essential and why promotion of antibiotic awareness now features in many clinical promotions and clinical treatment plans (Mitchell, 2015).

Antibiotic resistance

Antibiotic resistance is rising to dangerously high levels in all parts of the world with new bacterial resistance mechanisms emerging and spreading globally. This is threatening our ability to treat common infectious diseases such as pneumonia, tuberculosis, sepsis and gonorrhoea as antibiotics become much less effective. Campaigns from leading clinical institutions are directed at educating clinicians and the general public on the misuse of antibiotic treatments.

Further Reading

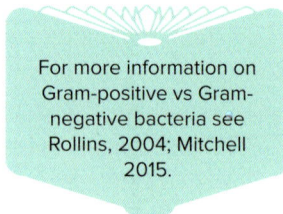

For more information on Gram-positive vs Gram-negative bacteria see Rollins, 2004; Mitchell 2015.

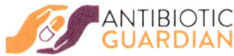

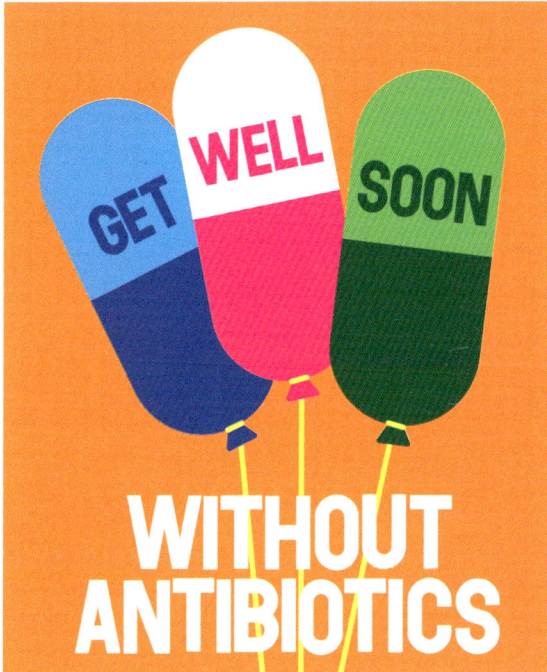

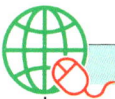

Useful Link

For more information on antibiotic resistance see Public Health England, 2018a: https://www.gov.uk/government/collections/european-antibiotic-awareness-day-resources.

Further Reading

For more information on antibiotics and their use see NHS Inform, 2019; WHO, 2018.

Ageing

As we age, our skin will change in appearance and function. As newborns, the adipose (fat) layers soon change from a heat- producing function (brown adipose) to an efficient energy source (white adipose), although the immature skin is not as efficient at regulating the surface temperature. Hormonal changes in our teenage years stimulate greater hair and oil production until we become elderly and our skin then becomes thinner which is once again not as efficient at dealing with surface temperature regulation.

Other contributing factors to skin degeneration:

- The regeneration of epidermal cells starts to reduce and so the epidermal layers become thinner.
- The dermis also becomes thinner in comparison to youthful dermal thickness as there are fewer collagen and elastic fibres present which in turn causes wrinkles and the skin to sag.
- Sweat glands become less active and less efficient at controlling our skin surface temperature.
- Less sebum production makes the epidermis very dry and flaky.
- Skin becomes much less effective at producing vitamin D from sunlight and this can lead to thinner and weaker bones.
- Melanocytes may become less active and so they cannot change the skin colour to protect us from harmful UV rays.
- Hair thins and becomes grey as the amount of melanin pigment becomes less and less.
- Hair also thins out in some areas but continues to prosper in more unwanted areas such as nose, ears, eyebrows in males and upper lips in females.

(MedlinePlus, 2019)

Ethnicity

Many examples of skin rashes referenced in textbooks are shown using examples on light skin. This is usually because the rash characteristics tend to be more prominent and easily seen in lighter skin, although examples which involve de-pigmentation are more easily seen in darker skin.

With the majority of skin conditions, the symptoms of itching, dryness and irritation are the same for all patients regardless of skin colour. It is worth considering that conditions such as changing moles and melanoma may be more difficult to see but will almost always be noticeable by the patient.

Cyanosis in darker skin presents as an ashen grey

- Check the lighter/pinker areas around the oral mucosa
- The conjunctivae may appear grey or bluish
- Capillary refill is likely to be delayed.

(Sommers, 2011)

Cyanosis or poor perfusion in lighter skin is again very easy to see and in some cases it can be quite a dramatic change.

Any skin type can develop scarring during the healing process so when the body over produces collagen around damaged sites, keloid scars can develop and spread into the surrounding healthy tissue.

Darker skin tends to have a higher risk of keloid scarring post-surgery or post-infection especially around the scalp, head and shoulders (NHS, 2019a).

Afro hair

The biochemical composition of Afro-textured hair is identical to that of Caucasians and Asians, although there are various classifications of Afro-textured hair which range from a looser curl texture to a tighter coil texture. It is the morphological difference in elasticity that causes Afro-textured hair to have different maintenance needs and potential development of clinical conditions.

- The tighter coils leave the hair more susceptible to breakage as combs and brushes force the curls to elongate, but the curls naturally resist which results in over-tressing of the follicles and breakage.

- Everyone's scalp naturally produces oily sebum fluid to moisturise and protect the hair follicle but the curliness of Afro-textured hair causes it to have less moisture content than other ethnic groups so additional oily hair products may be required. Both sebum and water travel down the hair shaft to lubricate the hair, but when these two elements are not able to travel all the way down the hair shaft or absorb into the hair strand, it leads to dry hair.

- The coiled shape of curly hair, does not create a straight path for sebum and water to travel all the way down the hair shaft and is why Afro-textured hair loses moisture quickly after washing. Washing hair daily will increase the risk of dryness.

(Loewenstein, 2016)

- Greater consideration needs to be taken into account when advising any clinical treatment regimens for afro hair. Washing twice weekly for instance with certain anti-fungal preparations may cause more damage to afro hair as it dries out.

(Sandeen, 2019)

Skin Healing and Wound Management

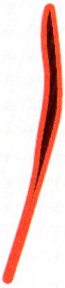

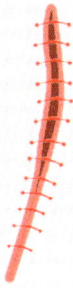

Wounds and the healing process

Wounds are injuries to living tissue which usually involve rupturing of the integument and mucous membranes to cause a division of tissues. The skin can be damaged by cutting, scraping, scratching, puncturing or from a direct blow during a traumatic event. Surgery, sutures and staples will cause an interruption to the blood supply and structures of the skin so are therefore also types of wounding. Wounds can be either open or closed and are classified depending on the mechanism of injury.

Open wounds

- **Incisions** result from surgery under sterile conditions where no organisms are present or by clean, sharp objects or cuts with sharp objects outside of theatre.
- **Abrasions** occur where the epidermis is scraped off causing a superficial wound.
- **Lacerations**, usually a result of blunt trauma, present as an irregular tear which may be linear (straight) or stellate (star-shaped) with the possibility of contamination by pathogens or foreign bodies being present in the wound.
- **Avulsions** are the forcible detachment of a structure from its normal insertion point, i.e. pulled off rather than cut off.
- **Puncturing** of the skin, usually with a long sharp object.
- **Penetration** is when an object such as a knife enters a sterile body cavity.
- **Infected** wounds occur where pathogenic organisms are present and multiplying within the wound which is also showing clinical signs of infection.
- **Colonised** wounds are a chronic wound containing pathogenic organisms delaying healing and are difficult to treat.

Incisions are often incorrectly classified as lacerations.

Closed wounds

- **Haematoma** – a collection of blood under the skin caused by damage to an underlying vessel
- **Crush injury** – caused by an extreme amount of force possibly over a prolonged period.

The three stages of wound healing

Although wound healing can be affected by both intrinsic and extrinsic factors which could lead to complications of healing, all wounds will follow a specific biochemical and cellular sequence which is both complex and multifactorial. There are three main stages of wound healing:

- **Inflammatory**
- **Proliferation**
- **Maturation.**

Useful Link

Watch how this works:
Wound healing: mode of action!

Coloplast, 2013:
https://www.youtube.com/watch?v=RiKu9sgFizY

The initial inflammatory phase is characterised by redness, swelling, heat and pain around the wound so it is important not to confuse this phase with the signs of infection. The inflammatory phase can last from 3 to 7 days depending on the damage to the injured tissues.

The inflammatory phase is vital for the healing process and is the reason why **non-steroidal anti-inflammatory medications should not be given in the first 48 hours post-injury.**

The inflammatory phase

- Mast cells de-granulate and release inflammatory mediators immediately after the wound occurs.
- This release causes local blood vessels to dilate.
- Neutrophils then digest bacteria in the wounded area.
- Flooding of the wound bed by macrophages follows which causes growth factors and prostaglandins to be released, influencing the healing process (Baxter, 2003).

The proliferation phase

- Growth of new vessels and tissue occurs during a reconstructive or proliferation phase of healing.
- Fibroblasts accumulate in the area and produce collagen. Collagen synthesis takes place alongside the growth of new vessels filling the wound with granulation tissue.
- Epithelial tissue forms at the edges of the wound while the wound contracts and the deficit is filled.
- This process continues until the wound is fully closed (Baxter, 2003).

The maturation and remodeling phase

- The maturation phase, also known as the remodeling stage, is the final phase of wound healing.
- The tensile strength of the wound is regained and the collagen fibres are re-organised so that the scar will lie flatter to the skin and lose some of the red pigmentation.
- This stage can take up to 18 months (Baxter, 2003).

Bleeding

Blood clot

Inflammatory

Scab

Fibroblast

Macrophage

Blood vessel

Proliferative

Fibroblasts proliferating

Subcutaneous fat

Remodeling

Freshly healed epidermis

Freshly healed dermis

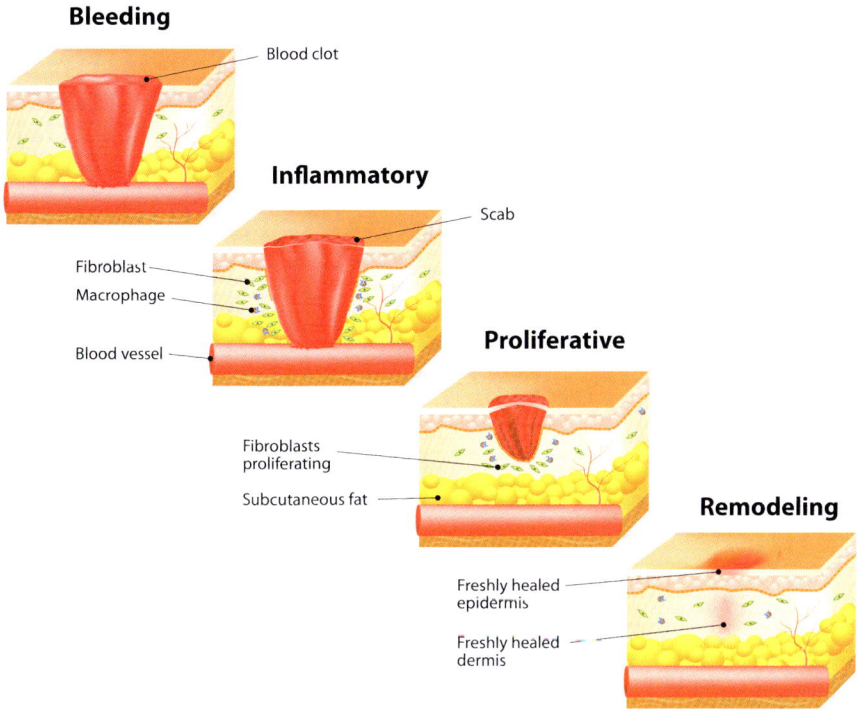

The prognosis for wound healing depends on the type of wound, any underlying injury and the baseline health of the patient. It is therefore a very individualised process which cannot always be predicted at the time of injury.

Cleaning the wound

If the wound is dirty, too old or it is thought there may be other reasons whereby closing of the wound would be inappropriate the wound may be allowed to heal by **secondary intention**. The wound would still be dressed regularly with continuous assessment but allowed to heal gradually over time without primary closure.

Potable water or normal saline are suitable for the cleansing of wounds although an aseptic technique will be required for immuno compromised patients and wounds which have entered a sterile body cavity.

- Primarily, the objective of wound cleansing is to remove foreign materials and reduce the risk of infection by lowering the bioburden. The bioburden is the number of bacteria which are contaminating an object.
- Materials that could potentially leave fibres in the wound, such as cotton wool, should not be used for the cleaning of wounds.

If a wound is properly cleaned and cared for there should be no reason to prescribe antibiotics. However, antibiotics may be prescribed prophylactically for significantly dirty wounds, animal bites or human bites, wounds that have been exposed to contamination by lake or river water. There is no evidence to support the use of topical antibiotics or any other creams/ointments to prevent wound infection. Indeed, antibiotic creams can cause irritation to the skin causing contact dermatitis, delay skin healing and greatly increase the risk of antibiotic resistance.

Further Reading

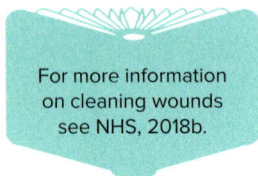

For more information on cleaning wounds see NHS, 2018b.

Use your clinical judgement to assess the risk of infection before considering closure!

Dressings

Use of dressings

Many dressings will need a retention bandage to keep them in place as repeated removal of adhesive dressings may damage the outer layer of the skin surrounding the wound, especially if the patient is elderly and the skin is fragile. The extent of damage is dependent on how much the dressing sticks to the wound or the adhesive sticks to the surrounding skin.

When a dressing is allowed to dry out it may stick to the wound or periwound skin. Removing a dressing which has become stuck to the wound may cause damage to newly formed, delicate wound tissue and surrounding skin causing severe pain. It is therefore important to select a dressing which can be left in situ for a number of days without causing trauma to the surrounding skin (Wounds International, 2013).

- Dressings stuck to skin should be soaked off with water
- Reducing pain when removing dressings is one of the factors which must be considered when choosing dressing materials.

The type of wound, location of wound, amount of exudate, patient skin condition, presence/absence of infection, condition of the wound bed, characteristics of the available dressings and treatment goals must influence the choice of dressing.

Strike through: Evidence of wound exudate appearing on the outer surface of the wound dressing indicating a need for dressing change.

Exudate saturating: Non-occlusive dressing which does not have a bacterial barrier is believed to act as a portal for the entrance of pathogens.

All dressings used in the management of wounds should be used in accordance with the manufacturer's instructions.

Types of dressings

Soft silicone dressings

Silicone dressings are part of the solid silicone family and cannot be absorbed by the body, which makes them ideal for wound dressings. These dressings are soft and tacky as they are coated with a hydrophobic soft silicone layer which allows them to conform and adhere gently to dry surfaces but not stick to moist wound beds, making removal non–traumatic to the wound or periwound skin. Soft silicones have low toxicity making the chance of adverse reactions rare (Wounds International, 2013).

Dressings which incorporate soft silicone have various target functions depending on the clinical need. These include: A wound contact layer to be used with a secondary dressing to decrease disruption to the wound bed, increasing patient comfort

- Absorbent dressings for moderately to highly exudating wounds
- As a first-line treatment of wounds at risk of keloid or hypertrophy scarring.

The dressing should be left in situ for at least 5 days. Burns require review within 48 hours (NICE, 2017b).

Soft silicone dressings should not be applied to wounds that are bleeding or patients with a known silicone allergy

The wound contact layers form a gentle seal between the dressing and the wound and is designed to allow exudates to pass through to an absorbent secondary layer. This ensures the fluid is taken up by the secondary part of the dressing and does not leak onto the surface of the skin. Such dressings have been shown to draw fluid vertically with no lateral movement of exudate onto the surrounding skin while an adhesive layer does not come into contact with the wound.

Soft silicone can be used on a wide range of low to highly exudating wounds. As it will remain tacky it stays in place ensuring wear times are longer which benefits healing, patient comfort and the use of healthcare resources.

Alginate dressings

Highly absorbent biodegradable alginate dressings contain sodium. They have been applied to successfully cleanse a wide variety of secreting lesions. Strong hydrophilic gel formation achieves high absorption, limits wound secretion and reduces bacterial contamination. Any alginate fibres that become trapped in the wound are readily biodegraded. A physiologically moist microenvironment is maintained by the alginate dressing which promotes the formation of new granulation tissue and thereby healing (Aderibigbe, 2018).

These dressing are suitable for moderate to heavy drainage wounds but not recommended for dry wounds, third degree burn wounds and severe wounds with exposed bone (Dhivya, 2015). They are useful for sloughy wounds which produce a degree of exudate and moderately to highly exudating wounds. The gel that is formed as a result of the absorption of the exudate prevents the slough from drying out as it forms a moist covering over the wound.

> **Alginate dressings are hydrophilic dressings which can absorb large volumes of exudate and maintain a moist wound interface without maceration of the skin.**

Alginates can be rinsed away with saline solution so healing tissue is not damaged during removal. Dressing changes are therefore virtually painless.

Hydrocolloids

These dressings have a unique design with interactive gel-forming agents which become active when in contact with a wound surface.
They are usually formulated with a water-repellent occlusive backing which promotes an acidic and hypoxic wound environment facilitating the development of new blood vessels (angiogenesis).

The dressing aims to promote an insulated moist healing environment while using the body's own enzymes to keep the wound bed hydrated.

The advantages of using hydrocolloid dressings are:

■ Easy to apply

■ They do not adhere to the wound site

■ They can be used with venous compression products

■ They are water repellent and only need to be changed after several days

■ They cause minimal disruption to the wound bed.

(Advanced Tissue, 2014)

The disadvantages of using hydrocolloid dressings are:

■ They are not indicated for high exudate, infected wounds or wounds with sinus tracking

■ There may be hyper-granulation and the skin around the wound can macerate

■ They are opaque (non-transparent) which makes assessment of the wound bed more difficult.

(Advanced Tissue, 2014)

Povidone iodine-impregnated dressings

These dressings are frequently used for a large variety of wound presentations as the iodine reduces any bacterial loading on the skin surface. In the presence of heavy exudate however, the antibacterial properties are rapidly exhausted and so they will need changing more frequently. This is signified when the orange dressing becomes white.

Transparent film dressings

These dressings promote **autolytic debridement** (selective to necrotic tissue) through maintaining a moist environment. They also function as a second skin by acting as a blister roof while protecting the wound from bacterial invasion and mechanical trauma.

> Transparent film dressings may be useful:
> - When intact skin needs protecting
> - To promote eschar debridement which is the product of the natural healing process
> - To secure another dressing
> - For use on partial thickness wounds with no or minimal exudate.

Transparent film dressings should not be used for patients with fragile or thin skin, especially elderly patients or those on long term steroid therapy, as removal can cause epidermal stripping.

The adhesive properties of these dressings are deactivated by moisture so they will not stick to a wound. They are also useful in suspected bacterial infections, fungal infections or active herpetic lesions. However, care needs to be taken as these dressings can lead to maceration of the skin (Morgan, 2014).

Closure and sutures

Wound closure

⚑ **Wounds with areas of high tension or repetitive movement should not be closed using skin adhesive or skin tapes.**

Once the decision has been made to close a wound this may be achieved by a number of different techniques:

- Suturing
- Surgical staples
- Skin closure tapes
- Adhesives
- Skin tying can sometimes be an option with partial thickness scalp wounds.

Sutures and skin adhesives have similar cosmetic outcomes and infection risks for minor or partial thickness lacerations <5cm in adults and children (Buchweitz, 2016).

Sutures

There are three types of suturing techniques used to close skin wounds:

- **Intermittent**
- **Blanket**
- **Continuous subcutaneous.**

Which one to use is dependent on the location of the wound, thickness of the skin, amount of tension in the wound and desired cosmetic effect.

- **Absorbable sutures**
  These breakdown in the tissues. They do not need removal.
- **Non-absorbable sutures**
  These do require removal.

> **If a wound is left open for longer than 6–8 hours it may not be sutured as the risk of infection increases over time.**

Removal of sutures

Before any sutures are removed the wound must be assessed as many factors will influence wound healing, making it an individual process for each patient. Suture removal depends on how well the wound is healing and the extent of surgery so they need to be left in situ long enough to establish wound closure with enough strength to support underlying internal structures.

- Facial sutures can be removed after 5 days
- Most other sutures can be removed at 7 days
- Sutures in wounds over 5 cm or over joints should remain in situ for 10–14 days.

(Holmes, 2019)

The longer the sutures remain in situ the greater the scarring.

Patients must be advised to keep sutures clean and dry as water can enter the skin through the suture wound itself and track down the suture causing an infection below the bed of the wound.

Alternate sutures are typically removed first with the rest of sutures being removed once adequate approximation of the skin and strength of the wound line has been determined. If the wound is well healed the remaining sutures can also be removed, but sometimes the remaining sutures can remain until days or even weeks later.

The wound line must be observed for any separation of the skin during the whole suture removal process.

If at any time it is noticed that the wound edges are opening, stop removing sutures and place adhesive strips over the wound line using tension to bring wound edges back together.

Remove every other suture until the end of the suture line is reached.

Removal of intermittent sutures

Remove any dressings and assess the wound for healing, any signs of infection or obvious ruptures along the surgical incision line known as **dehiscence**.

1. Clean wound line according to local policy

2. Remove alternate sutures by holding scissors/suture cutter in dominant hand and forceps in non-dominant hand

3. Place gauze or a gallipot close to the wound

4. Grasp the knot of the suture with the forceps and lift gently upwards while slipping the tip of the scissors/suture cutter under the knot close to the skin

5. Examine the knot to ensure it is intact

6. Cut under the knot as close to the skin as possible

7. Continue to grasp knotted end with the forceps and with one continuous movement pull the suture out of the skin and place on gauze or in gallipot.

Removing blanket sutures

- Repeat steps 1–5 as for intermittent suture removal
- Cut the first suture close to the skin surface distal to the knot.
- Cut the second suture on the same side
- Grasp knotted end with forceps and gently pull out suture
- Place suture on gauze or in gallipot
- Continue cutting in the same manner until the entire suture is removed, inspecting the wound line during the process.

Removal of continuous subcutaneous sutures

Most subcutaneous continuous sutures are absorbable, however, in some cases non-absorbable suture material may be used. Usually there will be a bead or other anchoring device visible on the skin at each end of the suture.

- Clean the skin underneath one of the beads
- Grasp the bead with the forceps
- Cut the suture close to the skin distal to the bead
- Grasp the other bead at the other end of the suture line with the forceps and pull the bead gently and horizontally along the skin in one slow continuous movement.

The whole suture will pull through the tissues attached to the bead.

Never pull contaminated suture material through the tissues.

Describing Skin Conditions

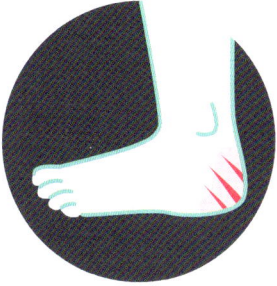

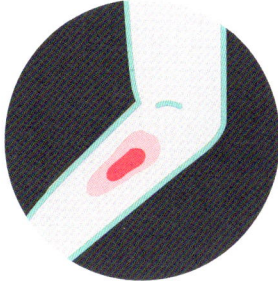

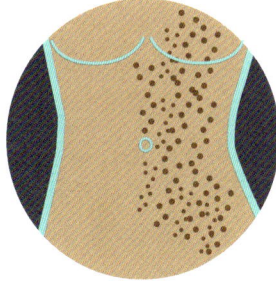

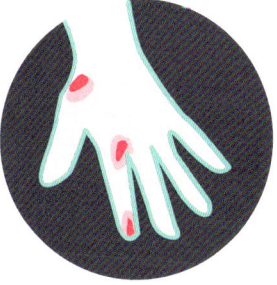

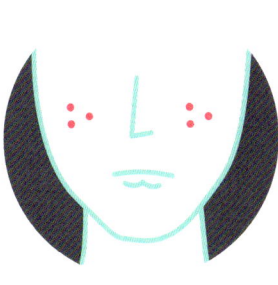

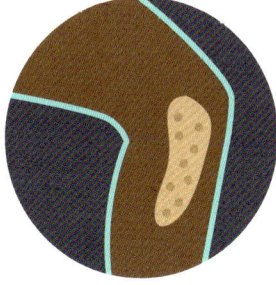

Why is terminology important?

Understanding descriptive terms for rashes and using them in documentation is obviously very important for continuity of accurate clinical notes and for an accurate diagnosis. If a patient with a rash requires referring to a specialist then using the correct descriptive terms adds to professional credibility.

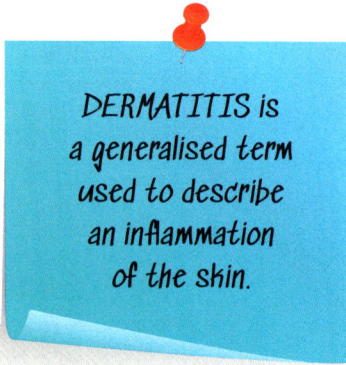

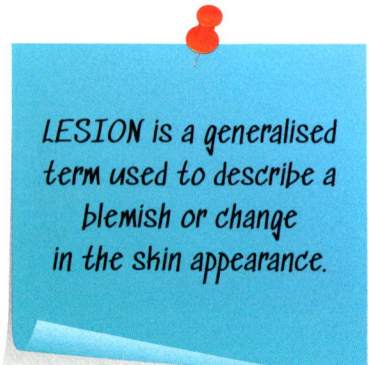

> DERMATITIS is a generalised term used to describe an inflammation of the skin.

> LESION is a generalised term used to describe a blemish or change in the skin appearance.

Describing surface changes

Scaly – covered by flakes

Wet/oozing – the water barrier of the skin is damaged and flow from beneath keeps the lesion wet

Crusted – dried serum

Excoriated – a lesion which has been scratched

Lichenified – a thickening of the epidermis with exaggeration of the normal skin lines.

Descriptive terminology

Atrophy – a thickness of substance of the epidermis or dermis

Blister – raised lesion containing fluid

Comedo – blackhead or blocked hair follicle

Cyst – deeper tissue swelling filled with fluid of a semi-solid matter

Eczematous – inflammation of the skin

Erosion – a partial loss of epidermis

Fissure – a crack or split in the epidermis

Lipoatrophy – a loss of subcutaneous fat

Lichenified – thickened, hard, leathery skin

Macule/Patch – a colour change of the skin only with no elevation (with your eyes closed this would not be felt at all)

■ Macule is less than 1cm. Patch is greater than 1 cm.

Papule/Nodule – a raised spot on the skin surface. Nodules are greater than 5 mm

Papulosquamous – papules or plaques with scale such as psoriasis, pityriasis rosea and secondary syphilis

Petechiae/Purpura – a purple discolouration of the skin caused by blood vessels (a common type is Henoch-Schonlein Purpura)

■ Petechial is less than 5 mm. Purpura is more than 5 mm.

Plaque – a raised, uniform thickening of skin with a well-defined edge and flat, rough surface

Pustule – skin filled with pus

Ulcer – a total loss of epidermis

Vesicle/Bulla – a fluid-filled blister

■ Vesicle is less than 5 mm. Bulla is more than 5 mm

Wheal – a transient pink plaque caused by oedema usually during urticarial rash.

Fissure

A crack or split in the epidermis

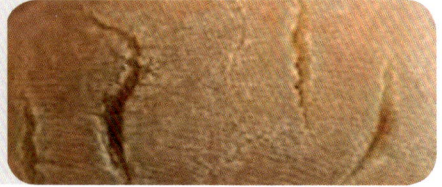

Macular rash

A colour change of skin only with no elevation evident

- A macular rash is less than 1 cm
- A patch is greater than 1 cm

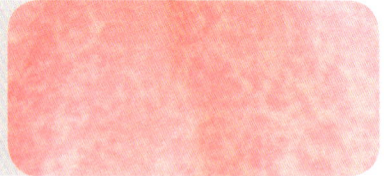

Papulosquamous

Papules or plaques with scale such as: psoriasis or pityriasis rosea

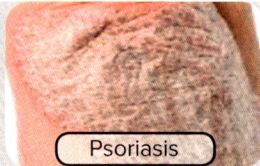

Psoriasis

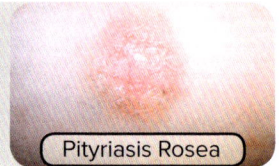

Pityriasis Rosea

Papule/nodule

A raised spot on the skin surface

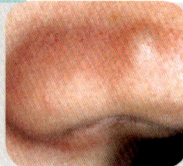

A nodule is greater than 5cm

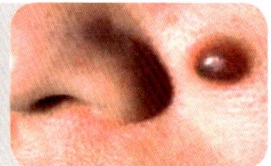

Petechiae/purpura

A purple discolouration of the skin caused by rupture of the blood vessels

Henoch-Schönlein purpura (HSP)
Children present with rash to lower limbs/calves and abdominal pains and possible haematuria

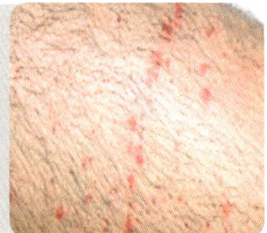

Skin plaque

A raised, uniform thickening of skin with a well-defined edge and flat, rough surface

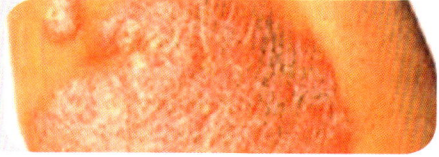

Pustule rash

Skin filled with pus

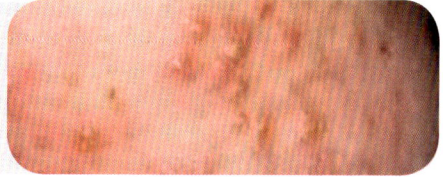

Ulceration

A total loss of the epidermis

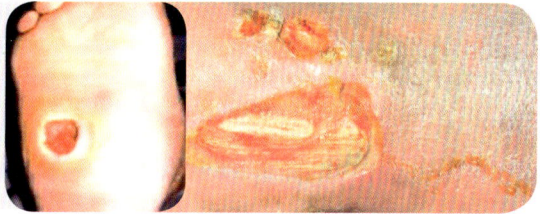

Vesicle/bulla

A fluid–filled blister

Vesicle – less than 5cm

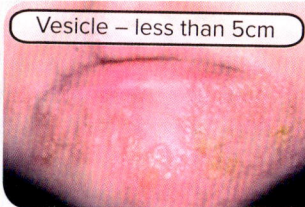

Bulla – more than 5cm

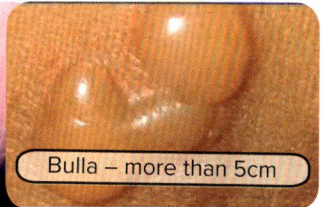

Wheal

A transient pink plaque caused by oedema usually during urticaria

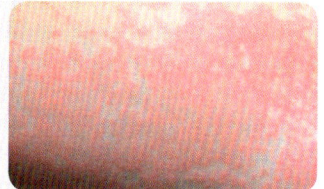

Terminology used in nail disorders

Leukonychia – white discolouration of the nail plate

Longitudinal ridges – the presence of lines or ridges that run along the length of the nail

Melanonychia – black or brown pigmentation of the nail plate

Onycholysis – detachment of the nail from the nail bed

Paronychia – inflammation and infection of the nail fold

Pits – punctate surface depressions in the nail plate, more commonly affecting fingers than toes

Pterygium – triangular formation of tissue within the nail

Subungual hyperkeratosis – excessive scaling under the nail

Transverse ridges – the presence of lines or ridges that run across the nail.

Further Reading

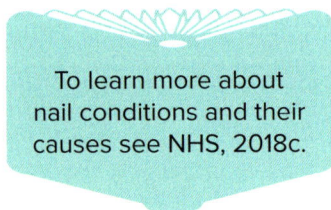

To learn more about nail conditions and their causes see NHS, 2018c.

Pharmacology

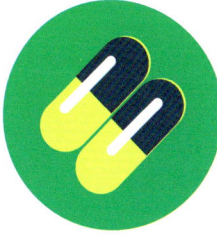

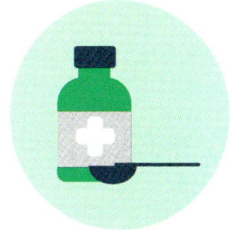

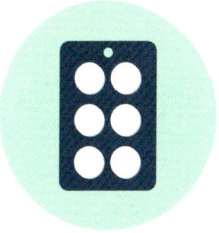

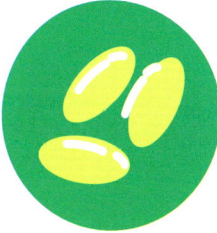

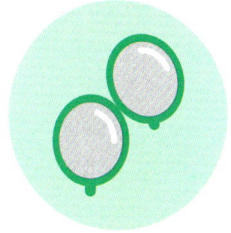

Emollients and moisturisers

Emollients and moisturisers help keep the skin moist and supple by reducing water loss from the epidermis, thereby providing a protective layer for patients with many varied skin conditions. The application of these products often forms an essential daily routine of skin care and is applied as often as necessary to control the condition.

Emollients are also found in many beauty applications such as lipsticks, lotions and cosmetic products, although general medical advice is to avoid these products especially with regards to severe skin conditions or acute exacerbation of dermatitis. There is a vast number of different emollients available which can be medicated or non-medicated but they include occlusive agents, lubricants, and humectants.

Emollients have a three-fold mechanism of action.

Occlusion	Humectant	Lubricant
Occlusive agents coat the skin forming a physical barrier that prevents the loss of water. Petroleum gel, waxes, oils and silicones are some examples. Individually, they can cause irritation on the skin so they are usually combined with another type of emollient.	**Humectants** include ingredients such as glycerin, urea and pyrrolidine carboxylic acid. They attract water from the atmosphere and also from the lower layers of skin to moisturise the skin surface. They can feel sticky so again they will be combined with other elements.	A **lubricant** reduces the friction when anything rubs against the skin.

Emollient products will vary according to the ratio of oil, or lipid, to water. The balance of occlusive, humectant and lubricant will also determine the type of moisturiser and its effectiveness.

Lotions, creams and ointments are all a mixture of oil and water so emulsifiers are added to keep them combined. The difference between the three types of products is the composition of the oil and water mixture. Ointments are made up of at least 70% oil whereas lotions are made up of 70% water. Creams are in between the two.

- **Creams** contain a mixture of fat (lipids) and water making them feel light and cool to the skin. All creams contain preservatives so patients can become sensitive to them.
- **Ointments** do not contain preservatives but can be very greasy which gives the skin a shiny appearance. They are very effective at holding water within the skin making them ideal for very dry and thickened skin conditions such as psoriasis.
- **Lotions** contain more water and less fat than creams so are not very effective at moisturising the skin but are useful for application to hairy areas of the body.

Examples of common emollients

- **Aqueous cream**
- **Aveeno**
- **Balneum** – cream / bath oil
- **Cetraben** – cream / bath additive / lotion
- **Dermol 500** – lotion / bath additive / cream
- **Diprobase** – cream / lotion / bath additive
- **Doublebase**
- **E45** – variant preparations and anti-itch
- **Emulsifying ointment**
- **Hydromol** – ointment / cream / gel
- **Oilatum**
- **Paraffin BP**
- **Zerobase 11%.**

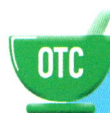

OTC

Most of these emollients are also available over the counter.

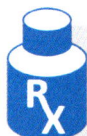

℞

These are often given as repeat prescriptions for patients too.

Quantity of emollients to prescribe

Emollient quantities according to the BNF (NICE, 2019c) are listed in the table below. These quantities represent sufficient amounts for a twice-daily application for a period of a week for an adult. Emollient should be applied as often as necessary to keep the skin soft and supple. The quantities required will vary with patient size, severity of the condition and the extent of the dryness (NICE, 2018b).

Body area	Creams and ointments	Lotions
Face	15–30 g	100 ml
Hands (both)	25–50 g	200 ml
Scalp	50–100 g	200 ml
Arms (both)	100–200 g	200 ml
Legs (both)	100–200 g	200 ml
Trunk	400 g	500 ml
Groin	15–25 g	100 ml

Tips for applying emollients

- Apply emollients and moisturisers daily especially after bathing while the water is still trapped in the skin
- Use at least twice a day but increase applications if the symptoms are not settling
- Apply gently and follow the direction of hair growth. Do not rub up and down as this can lead to itching, block hair follicles, and generate heat in the skin
- Continue to use the emollient after a flare-up has cleared as a preventative measure
- Non-medicated moisturisers are not harmful to the skin and most of these are safe during pregnancy or for paediatric use.

How much product do we apply?

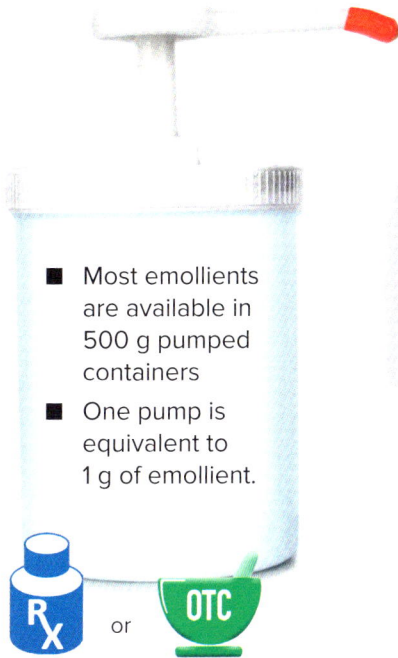

Face, neck
and ears **2 g**

Arms
2 g each

Torso
4–6 g

- Most emollients
are available in
500 g pumped
containers
- One pump is
equivalent to
1 g of emollient.

Hands
0.5 g for each

Cover for
both legs **8–9 g**

R X   or   OTC

Body area	Light dose	Medium dose	High dose
Arm	2 g (2 pumps)	5 g (5 pumps)	10 g (10 pumps)
Chest	2 g (2 pumps)	5 g (5 pumps)	10 g (10 pumps)
Abdomen	2 g (2 pumps)	5 g (5 pumps)	10 g (10 pumps)
Upper back	2 g (2 pumps)	5 g (5 pumps)	10 g (10 pumps)
Lower back	2 g (2 pumps)	5 g (5 pumps)	10 g (10 pumps)
Thigh	2 g (2 pumps)	5 g (5 pumps)	10 g (10 pumps)
Shin	2 g (2 pumps)	5 g (5 pumps)	10 g (10 pumps)

Further Reading

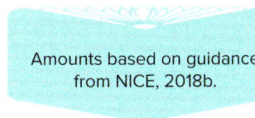

Amounts based on guidance
from NICE, 2018b.

Topical corticosteroids (steroids)

Corticosteroids (or steroids, as they are more commonly known) have been used for many years as a topical treatment for many kinds of inflamed skin conditions. Eczema is a prime example of this as the steroids can help reduce the unpleasant effects of redness, inflammation and

Consider hydrocortisone 1% in addition to emollients.

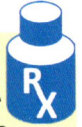

itching. They can be administered separately or as combinations of creams, ointments, lotions, gels and/or scalp applications which are widely available as branded or non-branded products. All of these are available on the NHS with a prescription. Some mild concentrations such as hydrocortisone 1% are available over the counter for the treatment of mild-to-moderate eczema which does not involve the face or genitals, although stronger concentrations are usually supplied under prescription for more severe cases (National Eczema Society, 2019).

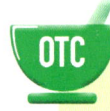

These are applied sparingly 2–3 times a day followed by an application of emollient on top each time.

It is important to consider that any application of topical steroids is avoided on open lesions due to the increased risk of wound infection and delayed healing.

Further Reading

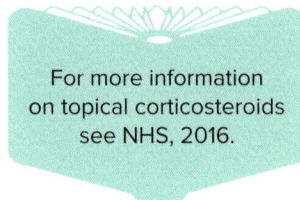

For more information on topical corticosteroids see NHS, 2016.

Topical corticosteroids are available in four potencies:

Mildly potent
- Hydrocortisone 0.1%, 0.5%, 1.0%, and 2.5%.

Moderately potent
- Betamethasone valerate 0.025% (Betnovate® RD)
- Clobetasone butyrate 0.05% (Eumovate®).

Potent
- Betamethasone valerate 0.1% (Betnovate®)
- Betamethasone dipropionate 0.05% (Diprosone®).

Very potent
- Clobetasol propionate 0.05% (Dermovate®)
- Diflucortolone valerate 0.3% (Nerisone® Forte).

Very potent topical corticosteroids should be prescribed by a doctor or specialist clinician.

Further Reading

Potency chart compiled using information from BAD, 2015; National Eczema Society, 2019; NHS, 2016a; NICE, 2019d.

Haelan® tape (fludroxycortide)

Haelan® tape is a thin, translucent dressing coated with an adhesive layer and contains a moderately potent corticosteroid called fludroxycortide. It must be used only on the skin (avoid eyes and mouth) and is generally applied for 12 hours a day but only for 5 days if using it for facial skin conditions.

Haelan® tape is very easy to apply and remains flexible so it's ideal for moving body parts such as hands, fingers etc. It is also waterproof making washing, showering and swimming more convenient for the patient, as well as having a matt finish to allow them to cover it with make-up if required (Online Clinic, 2019).

Tips for application

- Clean and dry the affected skin area

- Cut the Haelan® tape with clean scissors (it cannot be torn), ensuring it covers all the affected area with an all-round overlap of 0.5 cm onto unaffected skin

- Round off the square edges to prevent it sticking to clothes

- Remove the paper backing and stick the adhesive side of the translucent tape to the skin. Gently rub the tape from the middle to outer patch edges to ensure it sticks well

- Ensure to apply to flexed skin and bent joints so it does not become unstuck during daily activities

- Once applied, Haelan® tape must not be covered with another dressing or tight clothing.

(NICE, 2019e)

Eczema and Dermatitis

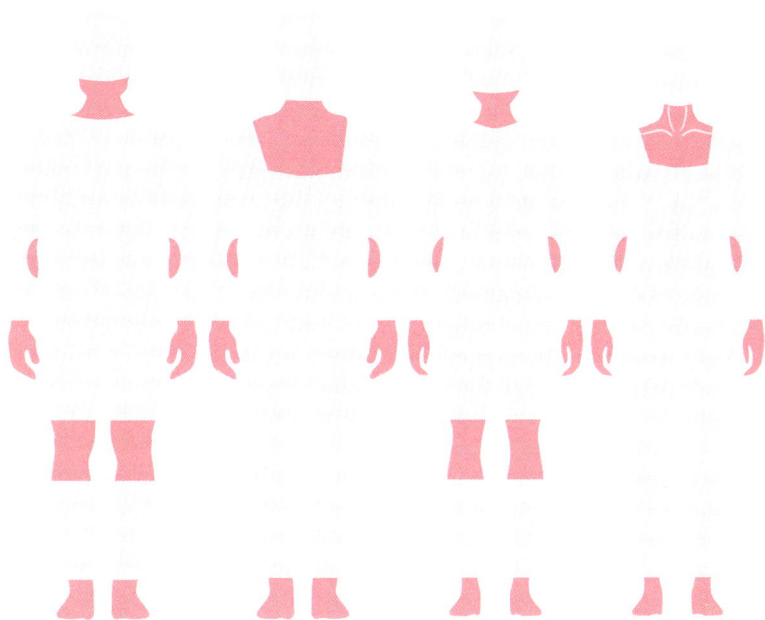

Atopic dermatitis and treatments

What is eczema?

Atopic dermatitis, commonly refered to as eczema, is a chronic skin condition that manifests itself with dry, scaly patches appearing on the skin. These patches are often intensely itchy although the symptoms can vary depending on the age of the patient. Most people develop atopic dermatitis before the age of 5 years and can continue to have symptoms as an adult (National Eczema Association, 2019a).

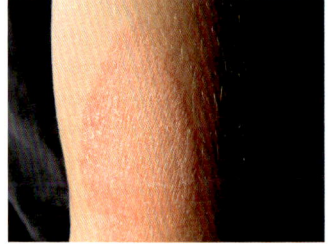

People with eczema will often experience periods where their skin will flare or worsen, followed by periods of time where their symptoms will improve or clear up. Symptoms can be exacerbated by some viral or bacterial infections, as well as other environmental factors and allergies.

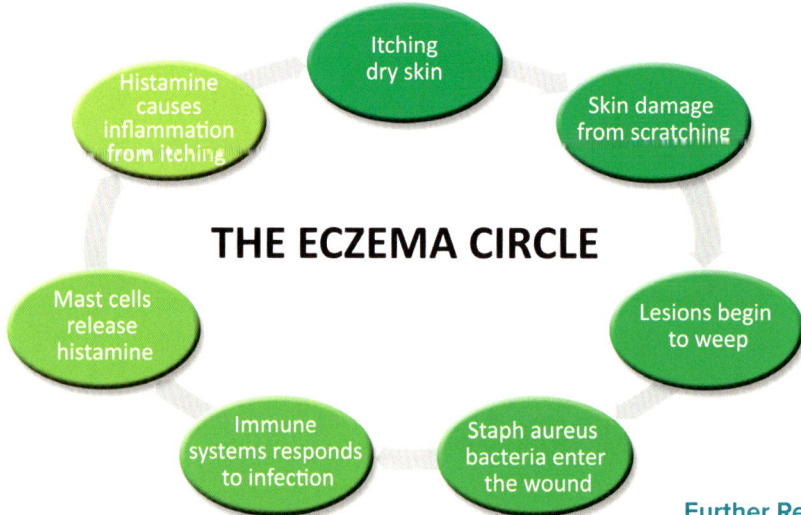

THE ECZEMA CIRCLE

- Itching dry skin
- Skin damage from scratching
- Lesions begin to weep
- Staph aureus bacteria enter the wound
- Immune systems responds to infection
- Mast cells release histamine
- Histamine causes inflammation from itching

Further Reading

For further information see NHS, 2019d; NICE, 2018b.

Treating eczema

One of the most important elements in managing all types of eczema is to keep the skin soft and supple by frequent and generous use of emollients (van Zuuren, 2017; Tucker, 2011).

Skin is thickest around the hands and feet and thinnest around the eyes so hydrocortisone is NOT recommend for eyelid applications.

Hydrocortisone 1% cream is often prescribed alongside emollients and is applied sparingly 2–3 times a day followed by an application of emollient on top each time.

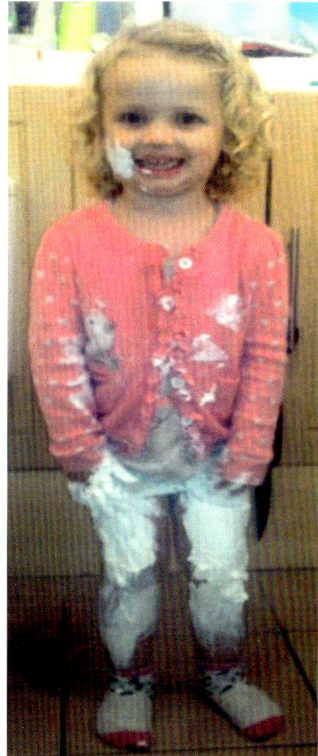

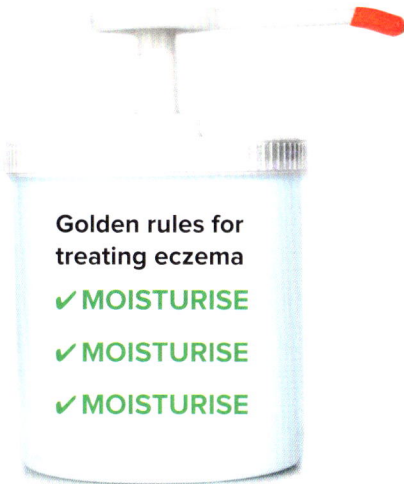

Golden rules for treating eczema

✔ MOISTURISE

✔ MOISTURISE

✔ MOISTURISE

NICE stepped treatment options for atopic eczema

The stepped approach, recommended by the National Institute for Health and Care Excellence (NICE, 2018b) for the treatment of atopic eczema, is shown below. Treatment can be stepped up or down according to the severity of the condition. Treatment of a flare will often require temporarily 'upping' the intensity of treatment (for example, the strength of corticosteroid).

Mild atopic eczema	Moderate eczema	Severe eczema
Emollients	Emollients	Emollients
Mild potency topical corticosteroids	Moderate potency topical corticosteroids	Potent topical corticosteroids
–	Topical calcineurin inhibitors (tacrolimus or pimecrolimus)*	Topical calcineurin inhibitors (tacrolimus or pimecrolimus)*
–	Bandages*	Bandages*
–	–	Phototherapy[†]
–	–	Oral corticosteroids[‡]

* Usually only prescribed by a specialist (for example, a GP with a specialist interest in dermatology, a dermatologist or a paediatrician).

[†] Phototherapy is available in secondary care for the treatment of very severe eczema that has proved resistant to standard treatment. Systemic immunosuppressants (for example, ciclosporin and azathioprine) are also available in secondary care for the same indication.

[‡] Oral corticosteroids can be prescribed short-term in primary care for severe flares. Other systemic treatments suitable for maintenance of severe eczema (for example, ciclosporin or azathioprine) require referral to secondary care.

- Topical calcineurin inhibitors, phototherapy and ciclosporin are less suitable for the acute treatment of flares
- Bandaging and oral corticosteroids are unsuitable for maintenance treatment.

Common sites of eczema

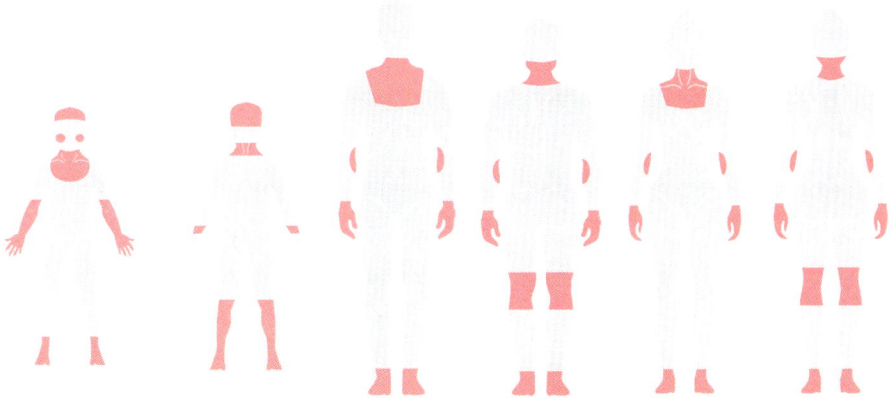

In children eczema commonly appears behind the creases of elbows or knees but may also affect neck, wrists, ankles and the crease between buttock and leg (National Eczema Association, 2019a).

Common eczema triggers
- Dry or cold climate
- Heat
- Stress
- Lack of important minerals such as zinc
- Exposing skin to harsh conditions
- Wool or synthetic material
- Certain detergents, soaps, cosmetics or perfumes
- Cigarette smoke
- Dust or mould
- Food allergies
- Hormonal changes.

(NHS, 2019b)

Other variants of eczema include:
- **Allergic contact eczema (dermatitis)** – a skin reaction following contact with an allergen that the immune system recognises as foreign
- **Discoid eczema** is a type of eczema that occurs in circular or oval patches on the skin. It is also known as nummular eczema
- **Seborrhoeic eczema** – oily, scaly, yellowish patches of skin, usually on scalp and face.

(National Eczema Association, 2019b)

Contact dermatitis

Contact dermatitis describes the inflammation that is caused by an irritant of some kind having contact with the skin surface. It is sometimes called contact eczema. One example of this is nickel metals found in jewellery or belt buckles touching the skin and causing a topical reaction (Harding, 2014; BAD, 2017a).

Symptoms

- Eczema-type presentation which can appear dry and possibly cracked
- Can also appear red and scaly with small blisters which leak fluid when scratched
- May be similar shape to object causing the irritation
- Deeper lesions can develop and become infected.

Emollients, barrier and 1% steroid creams are readily available **OTC**

Promote regular use of emollients to soothe and protect the skin preventing further problems (British Skin Foundation, 2019a).

Some of these are available over the counter (OTC) so check directory for costs and suitability.

Treatment

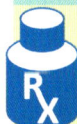

Check **BNF** dosage and local antimicrobial guidelines

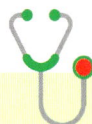

- ✔ Consider antihistamine medications but warn of the risk of drowsy side effects with some of these
- ✔ Hydrocortisone 1% or stronger steroid creams may be beneficial but do not apply to open wounds (NICE, 2018a)
- ✔ Consider Haelan® tape (PCDS, 2019a).

- Most obvious treatment is to remove the irritant if possible
- Avoid scratching
- Initially wash the hands in warm water to remove any possible residue
- Treatment plans should focus around prevention of contact and regular moisturising and use of barrier creams (NICE, 2018a).

Any lesions with exudate may require a swab to be sent to check for secondary infections.

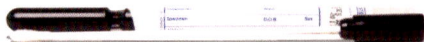

Discoid eczema

Discoid eczema is also known as nummular or discoid dermatitis and is a chronic skin condition that can keep recurring in the same areas with symptoms lasting months or years. It usually occurs in adults, particularly middle aged men, with no previous history of skin disease. It can be seasonal and worsens in winter but improves in summer (AAD, 2019).

Symptoms

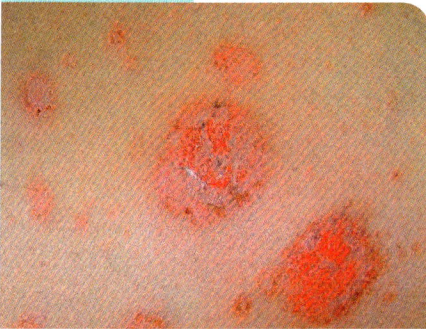

The condition presents as a well demarcated circular or oval patch which affects any part of the body causing the skin to become itchy, inflamed and cracked.

Further Reading

For full details see PCDS, 2016a. The Primary Care Dermatology Society also offers a wealth of resources on other skin conditions.

Treatment

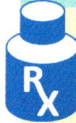

Check **BNF** dosage and local antimicrobial guidelines
✔ Emollients
✔ Topical steroids creams are very effective and should be prescribed along with emollients
NOTE: mild steroids initially, but may require a more potent steroid if the condition is not settling
✔ Consider a steroid-antibiotic combination such as betamethasone valerate + clioquinol (Betnovate® C)
✔ Consider Haelan® tape.

A combination of all treatments may be effective since secondary infection with Staphylococcus aureus in adults is common.

(BAD, 2019a; NICE, 2018b; PCDS, 2016a)

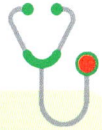

Seborrhoeic dermatitis

Symptoms

Seborrhoeic dermatitis is actually a form of eczema and appears on the body where there is a greater quantity of oil-producing (sebaceous) glands such as the shoulders and upper back, around the nose and over the scalp. In adolescents and adults seborrhoeic dermatitis usually presents as scalp scaling and dandruff (NICE, 2019f).

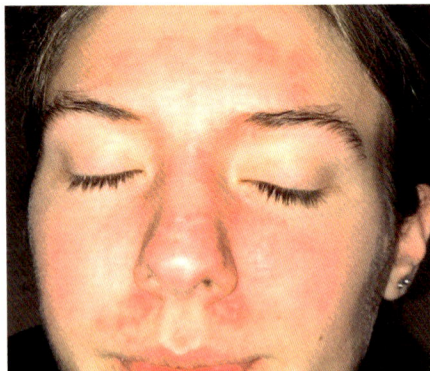

Common features include:

Inflammation – greasy skin – white or yellow crusty flakes

In infants, seborrhoeic dermatitis is known as cradle cap. Parents will often become concerned about when it appears but most cases will clear up after a few months without the need for treatment (NICE, 2019f).

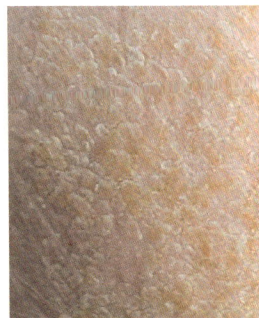

Treatment

Topical antifungal medications or shampoo such as **ketoconazole** or **miconazole** are effective treatments for seborrhoeic dermatitis and dandruff.

To help reduce the build-up of cradle cap, there are several treatment options:
- Soften the scales with baby oil first, alternatively soak the crusts overnight with white petroleum jelly or vegetable/olive oil
- Wash off with baby shampoo followed by gentle brushing.

(NICE, 2019f)

Psoriasis

Symptoms

Psoriasis is an incurable chronic autoimmune condition that results in the overproduction of the skin cells. The dead cells build up into silvery-white scales which can cause the skin to become more inflamed leading to a very uncomfortable itching sensation. Most cases of psoriasis go through cycles, causing problems for a few weeks or months before easing or stopping.

Psoriasis can appear anywhere on the body but common areas to be affected are:

- Elbows
- Knees
- Scalp
- Lower back.

(NICE, 2018c)

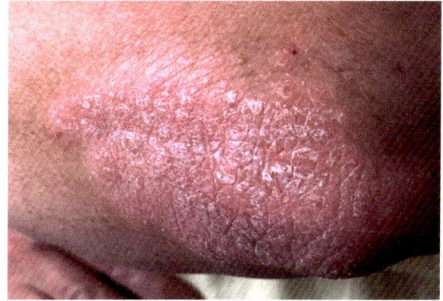

The (**papulosquamous**) plaques can be itchy, sore or both.

In severe cases, the skin around the joints may crack and bleed.

One of the most important factors to consider with patients suffering from psoriasis is the additional psychological effect this can cause. Some patients suffer with exacerbated anxiety or depression with flares of psoriasis that can lead them to feel extremely self-conscious and isolated.

They may become reluctant to socialise or take part in sports because of how they visualise their own skin, and also feel a need to hide the condition from others.

Consider psychological effects for someone with psoriasis.

There are several different types of psoriasis with most patients suffering from one form at a time, but two different types of psoriasis can occur together or even grow into another type (NHS, 2018c).

- **Plaque psoriasis (psoriasis vulgaris)** is the most common form which produces the classic plaques covered in silver scales.

- **Scalp psoriasis** affects patches or the whole scalp presenting as red patches of skin covered in thick silvery-white scales. In some cases this can lead to temporary hair loss which again increases the psychological problems for some people.

- **Nail psoriasis** can cause the nails to develop unevenly and become discoloured. They may also become loose with severe cases causing the nail to become extremely brittle. Acropustulosis causes pustules to appear on the fingers and toes. The pustules then burst, leaving bright red areas that may ooze or become scaly and can lead to painful nail deformities.

- **Inverse (flexural) psoriasis** affects the natural folds in the skin such as the armpits, groin, buttocks and under breasts. It can cause large, smooth, red patches in some or all of these areas. Affected areas will be exacerbated by friction and sweating, making it much worse in hotter climates. Not to be confused with intertrigo.

- **Guttate psoriasis** causes small (less than 1 cm) sores on the chest, arms, legs and scalp. Most cases will resolve after a few weeks although some patients may go on to develop plaque psoriasis

- **Palmoplantar pustular psoriasis** causes pustules to recurrently appear every few days or weeks on the palms of the hands and soles of the feet. The pustules gradually develop into circular brown, scaly spots which then peel off.

Treatment

Managing psoriasis depends on the severity of the condition and which area of the body is affected. Support for anxiety or depression should also be considered. Generally, emollients or lotions are given as a primary treatment plan (NICE, 2018c).

Vitamin D preparations

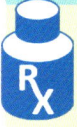
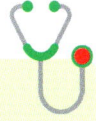

Topical vitamin D preparations are available as ointments, gels, scalp solutions and lotions. Three vitamin D preparations are available on prescription in the UK:

Calcipotriol (Dovonex®) — available as an ointment

Calcipotriol (non-branded) — available as an ointment and scalp solution

Calcitriol (Silkis®) — available as an ointment

Tacalcitol (Curatoderm®) — available as an ointment or lotion

Note: calcitriol and tacalcitol may be less irritating than calcipotriol.

(ABPI, 2019; BNF, 2017)

Salicylic acid

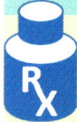
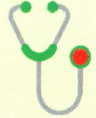

Products suitable for the scalp include:

Sebco® scalp ointment
(coal tar 12%, salicylic acid 2%, sulphur 4%, coconut oil)

Psorin® scalp gel (dithranol 0.25%, salicylic acid 1.6%)

Capasal™ shampoo (coal tar 1%, coconut oil 1%, salicylic acid 0.5%)

Meted® shampoo (salicylic acid 3%, sulphur 5%)

Products suitable for plaques on the trunk and limbs include:

Zinc and salicylic acid paste (Lassar's paste: zinc oxide 24%, salicylic acid 2%)

Psorin® ointment (dithranol 0.11%, coal tar 1%, salicylic acid 1.6%).

(BNF, 2017)

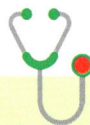

Coal tar products

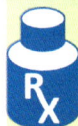

Several coal tar preparations are available in the UK including ointments, shampoos and bath additives. Various preparations are combined with other topical treatments for the management of psoriasis (for example salicylic acid).

The choice of coal tar preparation should take into consideration product availability, the skin site, previous response to treatment and the person's preference. Newer, branded products are preferred because older, non-branded products contain crude coal tar (coal tar BP) which is smellier and usually messier to use.

Preparations suitable for treating scalp psoriasis include:
Alphosyl® 2 in 1 shampoo (alcoholic coal tar extract 5%)
Capasal™ shampoo (coal tar 1%, coconut oil 1%, salicylic acid 0.5%)
Polytar® liquid shampoo (coal tar 4%)
Psoriderm™ — scalp lotion is also a shampoo (coal tar 2.5%, lecithin 0.3%)
T/Gel® shampoo (coal tar extract 2%)
Exorex® lotion (coal tar 5%)
Sebco® scalp ointment (coal tar solution 12%, salicylic acid 2%, sulphur 4%)
Note: do not use coal tar shampoos such as Polytar®, Alphosyl® 2 in 1, or Capasal® alone for treating severe scalp psoriasis.

Preparations suitable for treating psoriasis include:
Exorex® lotion (coal tar 5%)
Psoriderm™ cream (coal tar 6%)
Bath additives include:
Polytar Emollient® bath additive (coal tar solution 2.5%, peanut oil, extract of coal tar 7.5%, tar 7.5%, cade oil 7.5%, liquid paraffin 35%).
Psoriderm™ bath emulsion (coal tar 40%).

(BNF, 2017)

Fungal Infections

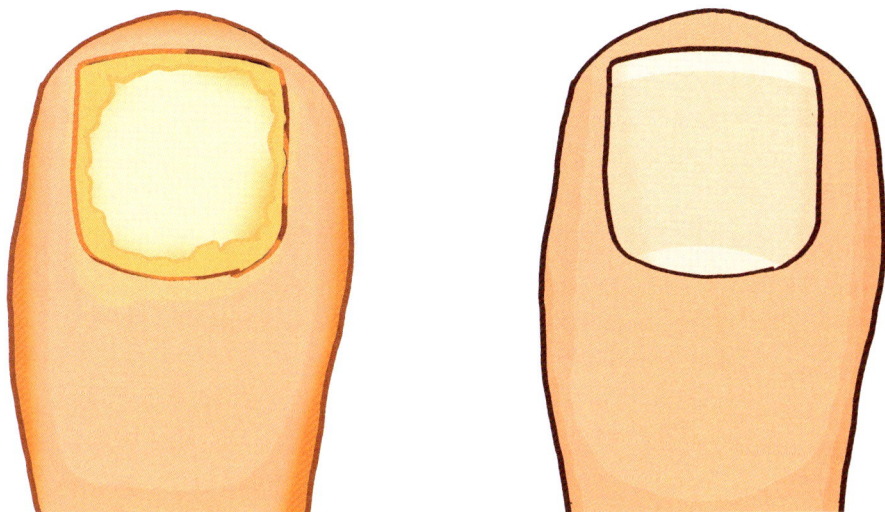

Tinea infections

Tinea is a common fungal infection caused by a dermatophyte fungi which requires keratin in order to grow (keratin is a protein that protects epithelial cells within the skin). A dermatophyte that survives on a human host is defined as an anthropophilic dermatophyte. Fungal infections are not usually serious and can be easily treated although treatment can take months to be completely effective. These infections are very contagious and easily spread from host to host by humans, animals or soil (Likness, 2011).

Symptoms

A tinea rash is usually asymmetrical and has a well-defined leading edge which is generally red or silver, rough or scaly and itching. They tend to grow outwards on the skin and form a ring-like pattern, hence the term **ringworm**.

The variations of tinea infections can be titled by their clinical appearance and on which part of the body they have infected.

- **Tinea corporis** (body)
- **Tinea cruris** (groin)
- **Tinea pedis** (feet)
- **Tinea manuum** (hands)
- **Tinea unguium** (nails)
- **Tinea capitis** (scalp)
- **Tinea faciei** (face)
- **Tinea versicolor** (skin).

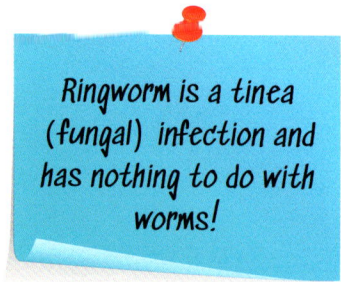

Ringworm is a tinea (fungal) infection and has nothing to do with worms!

Consider sending hair samples or skin scrapings for analysis. Hair follicles must include the bulb (root) not just a cutting (Dermapak, 2018).

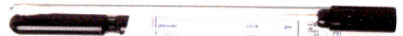

OTC Varied products available

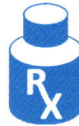

R℞ Check **BNF** dosage and local antimicrobial guidelines

Tinea corporis (body)

Treatment

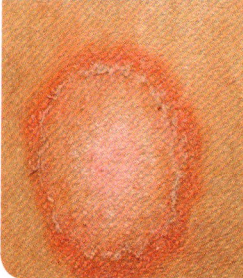

- ✔ **Clotrimazole 1%** apply 2–3 times a day and continue for at least 4 weeks
- ✔ **Miconazole 2%** apply 2 times a day and continue for 10 days after all skin lesions are healed
- ✔ **Econazole 1%** apply 2 times a day and continue until all lesions are healed
- ✔ **Terbinafine 1% topical/250 mg oral** (PCDS, 2017a).

Tinea capitis (scalp)

Treatment

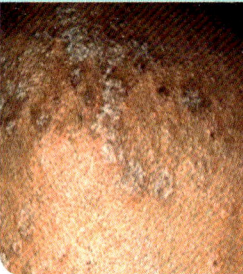

- ✔ **Ketoconazole 2% shampoo** adolescents and adults only
- ✔ **Selenium 2.5% shampoo** for adults and children aged 5 years+ (BAD, 2017b)
- ✔ **Terbinafine 1% topical/250 mg oral**
- ✔ **Itraconazole 10 mg oral solution or 100mg capsules** (PCDS, 2019b).

Tinea pedis (feet)

Treatment

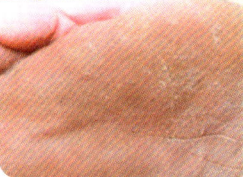

- ✔ **Clotrimazole 1% cream**
- ✔ **Miconazole 2% cream**
- ✔ **Undecenoic acid (Mycota®)**
- ✔ **Terbinafine 1% topical/250 mg oral** (Starr, 2018).

Tinea unguium (nail)

Symptoms

The terminology for a fungal nail infection is **onychomycosis**. Fungal infections of the nails are common and early signs of infection will cause the nail to become discoloured, thick and likely to split or break. Infections are generally more common in toenails than fingernails.

If left untreated, the skin underneath and around the nail can become inflamed and painful. There may also be white or yellow patches on the nailbed or scaly, dry, pungent skin next to the nail. Patients with onychomycosis may also suffer additional anxiety due to the appearance of the infection, especially with fingernails.

Some contributing risk factors to consider regarding history are:

- Ageing, poor peripheral circulation, poor nail growth and chronic or recurrent fungal infections all cause nails to grow slowly and increase the risk and problems of infections
- Diabetes
- Immunosuppressed patients
- Athlete's foot (Tinea pedis)
- Nail fungus tends to affect men more often than women
- Sweaty feet, humid or moist environment, poor shoe ventilation and walking barefoot in damp public places such as swimming pools (Mayo Clinic, 2019b).

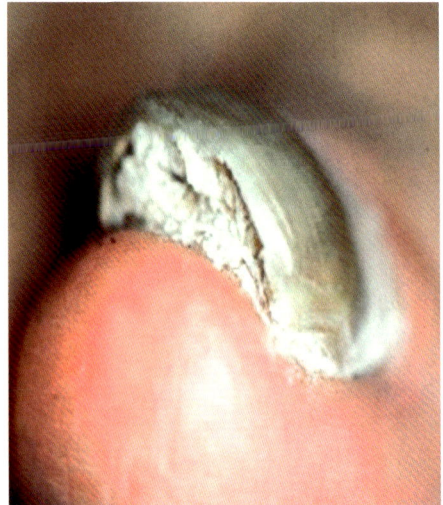

Consider sending nail clippings or skin scrapings for analysis in a **DERMAPAK**®

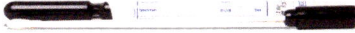

DERMAPAK® TYPE 4 FOR IN VITRO USE ONLY

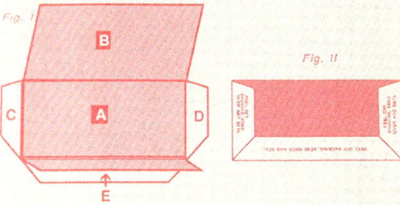

Fig. I

B

C | A | D

E

Fig. II

INSTRUCTIONS

Remove Dermapak from outer resealable plastic bag.

Lift top cover (B) and place specimen centrally onto base (A) [see Fig I].

Gently lower cover (B) onto specimen.

Peel off backing from self-adhesive side flaps (C,D&E).

Seal Dermapak by folding over flaps and attaching them to front cover [see Fig II].

Complete the information requested on label (1,2,3,4,5 & 6).

Replace Dermapak into resealable plastic bag and send to Laboratory with request form.

To prevent recurrence apply 1% topical antifungal cream to the entire area.
Children – seek specialist advice.

Further Reading

For more information take a look at NICE, 2018d.

Treatment

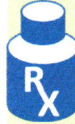

Check **BNF** dosage and local antimicrobial guidelines

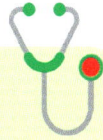

1st line
✔ Terbinafine 250mg OD (NICE, 2018d):
Fingers 6 weeks
Toes 12 weeks.

2nd line
✔ Itraconazole 250mg BD 1 week per month (NICE, 2018d):
Fingers 2 courses
Toes 3 courses.

If Candida or non- dermatophyte infection is confirmed then use oral itraconazole (NICE, 2018d).

- Take nail clippings
- Start therapy with confirmation of infection
- Oral terbinafine is more effective than oral azole
- Liver reactions 0.1–1% with oral antifungals
- Topical nail lacquer is NOT as effective.

Stop treatment when continual, new or healthy proximal nail growth
(NICE, 2018d).

Tinea versicolor

Symptoms

Pityriasis versicolor, also called tinea versicolor is a fungal infection caused by a type of yeast called Malassezia. This yeast is found on the skin of more than 90% of adults and normally lives without causing any problems (NICE, 2015).

When the yeast starts to multiply it appears as a rash on the skin. Because the yeast grows naturally on the skin it is not contagious but can affect people of any skin colour. It's more likely to affect teenagers and young adults (NICE, 2015).

Some contributing factors to stimulate the yeast to grow are (NICE, 2015):

- Living in a hot climate
- Sweating
- Oily skin
- Immunocompromised patients.

This isn't related to poor hygiene.

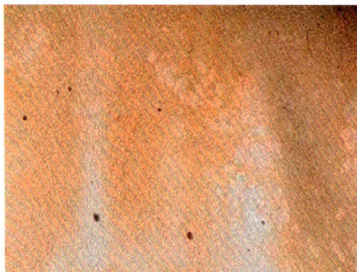

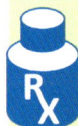

Treatment

Check **BNF** dosage and local antimicrobial guidelines

Itching symptoms may ease with antihistamine medication
OTC or prescription antifungal topical products containing:

- ✔ Miconazole
- ✔ Clotrimazole or selenium sulphide.

- Treatment consists of topical antifungal creams, lotions or shampoos
- Application of emollients may also help prevent any further dry skin conditions.

(NICE, 2015)

Discolouration of the skin may take up to several months to resolve

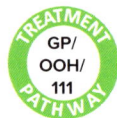
TREATMENT
GP/
OOH/
111
PATHWAY

Tinea cruris (jock itch)

Tinea cruris (jock itch) is a dermatophyte (fungal) infection of the skin which can develop quickly in warm, moist areas, especially around the groin, inner thighs and buttocks. This tends to be most common in men and adolescent boys but is typically a mild infection.

Symptoms

The infection causes an itching or burning type rash that can also be very red, flaky or scaly.

Note the risk of secondary infections

Monitor diabetic patients for infections

Consider swab and send for fungal culture

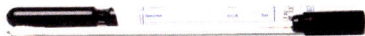

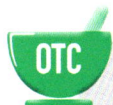

OTC Emollients, barrier creams, talcum powders, antifungal creams.

Treatment

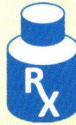

Check **BNF** dosage and local antimicrobial guidelines

✔ Topical treatment with antifungal creams such as **clotrimazole 1%** which may be combined with a steroid cream e.g. **trimovate**
✔ Topical or oral antibacterial treatment may also be indicated
✔ Antihistamine may help with itch.

(NICE, 2018e)

Patient advice includes:
- Drying the skin with talcum powder
- General hygiene
- Weight loss may be beneficial
- Also check for signs of athlete's foot.

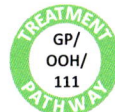

TREATMENT
GP/
OOH/
111
PATHWAY

Balanitis

Balanitis affects the head of the penis and the foreskin and can be caused by a bacterial or fungal infection such as thrush or by urine irritation. It occurs far more often in men and boys who haven't been circumcised. Consider history and any additional risk factors for sexually transmitted diseases (STD) in men or adolescents.

Symptoms

- Red swollen penis tip which can be sore and itchy
- Possible smelly discharge
- Build-up of thick fluid
- Pain when passing urine.

Urinary retention

**Check for glucose
Check for infection**

Send a urine specimen for culture and sensitivities

Swab and send for a fungal culture

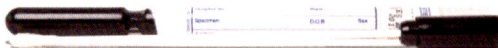

Treatment

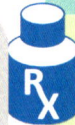

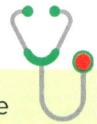

Check **BNF** dosage and local antimicrobial guidelines

Primary choice antibiotics for children:

✔ **Clotrimazole with hydrocortisone cream**

✔ **Flucloxacillin** if any cellulitis present

✔ **Clarithromycin** if penicillin allergy.

(NICE, 2018f)

- Advise gentle cleaning with warm water avoiding soaps
- Gently retract foreskin regularly to clean. May be difficult and require review if the foreskin is too swollen.

(NHS, 2017c)

Candidiasis

Candidiasis is a fungal infection caused by yeasts from the genus Candida which are a normal part of the commensal flora within the gastrointestinal tract and the vagina (NICE, 2017c). In fact, there are about 20 different species of Candida and the most common to cause infection in humans is Candida albicans (PCDS, 2016b).

Symptoms

Overgrowth of these yeasts leads to symptoms of dermal conditions/infections and they will vary depending on the area of the body that is affected.

- **Intertrigo** (skin fold infections) — commonly occurring in the groin, under the breasts, antecubital fossae (elbow creases), within the umbilicus, perineum, finger folds, neck creases and eyelids
- **Genital infections**
  - Vulvovaginal candidiasis
  - Balanitis: inflammation of the glans penis
- **Nappy rash** – dermatitis
- **Oral candidiasis** – infection of the oral mucosa/mouth/tongue.

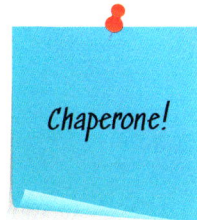

Consideration and documentation for a CHAPERONE is of paramount importance especially with genital or breast examinations. Check your surgery/walk-in centre or hospital policy for clarification.

Chaperone!

Treatment

Depending on your scope of practice, examination, diagnosis and treatment of genital infections may not be appropriate for some clinicians.

History taking may give an adequate indication of the problem but seeking further advice and support from a duty doctor or qualified clinician for treatment plans is strongly advised.

Oral candidiasis (thrush)

A fungal infection which is relatively common in babies or with patients who have inhaled steroids or are immunosuppressed (NICE, 2017d).

Symptoms

Thick white deposits are visible on the tongue and the roof of the mouth which is very hard to remove/scrape off. Milk deposits can sometimes be mistaken for oral thrush (NICE, 2017d).

Advice for application

With **breastfed babies** that are suffering with oral candidiasis (NHS, 2018e):

✔ The gel is best applied to the mother's nipples as well as the baby's mouth to prevent cross infection

✔ Wipe the breast clean prior to feeding and clean the breast post-feed before reapplying the antifungal treatment.

With patients using inhaled steroids:

✔ Advise the use of an Aerochamber

✔ Rinse mouth afterwards with water.

Treatment

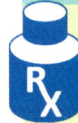

Check **BNF** dosage and local antimicrobial guidelines

Antifungal medications:

✔ **Miconazole oral gel**
Age 4 months+

✔ **Nystatin 100,000 units/ml oral suspension**
Age I month+

✔ **Oral fluconazole** in severe infections but discuss with duty doctor.

(NICE, 2017d)

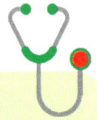

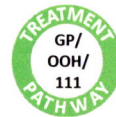

GP/
OOH/
111

Vaginal candidiasis

Candida species can multiply and cause an infection if the environment inside the vagina changes in a way that encourages their growth. This can happen because of hormones, medicines or changes in the immune system. Candidiasis in the vagina is commonly called a 'vaginal yeast infection'. Other names for this infection are vaginal thrush, vulvovaginal candidiasis or candida vaginitis. Women who are more likely to get vaginal candidiasis include those who:

- Are pregnant
- Use hormonal contraceptives (for example, birth control pills)
- Have diabetes
- Have a weakened immune system
- Are taking or have recently taken antibiotics (NICE, 2017e).

Symptoms

- Vaginal itching or soreness
- Pain during sexual intercourse
- Pain or discomfort when urinating
- Abnormal vaginal discharge
- Although most vaginal candidiasis is mild, some women can develop severe infections involving redness, swelling and cracks in the wall of the vagina.

Treatment

Most infections are treated with an antifungal medicine applied inside the vagina or a single dose of fluconazole taken orally (NICE, 2017e).

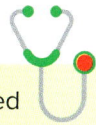

Consider:

- Dip stick urinalysis
- Pregnancy test
- History or risk of sexually transmitted disease (STD).

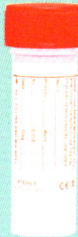

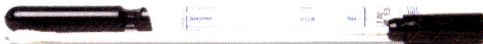

A swab of vaginal discharge is sent to a laboratory for a fungal culture to diagnose vaginal candidiasis as the symptoms are similar to those of other types of vaginal infections. A positive fungal culture does not always mean that Candida is causing the symptoms though as some women can have Candida in the vagina without having any symptoms.

Pityriasis rosea (Christmas tree rash)

As dramatic as this condition can appear, it is a self-limiting infection which causes a widespread blanching rash on the back and trunk.

It affects mainly adolescents and young adults although the actual cause of this reaction is still unknown (NICE, 2016a).

Symptoms

A larger **herald patch** is usually apparent within the first 2 weeks before a larger eruption of small patches is seen. Their appearance is a variant ring scaling formation. Patches along the dermatome lines will appear as the Christmas tree pattern (NICE, 2016a).

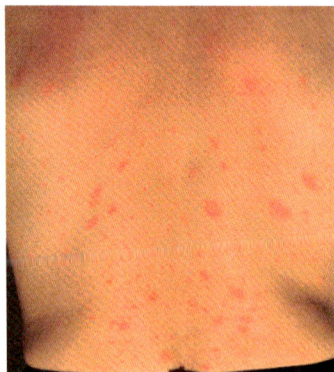

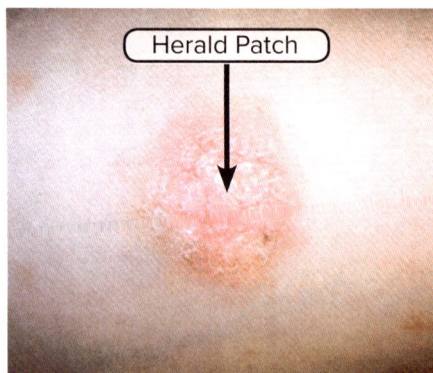

Herald Patch

Treatment

This can take several months to clear completely but does not require specific medication (NICE, 2016a). Application of emollients may also help prevent any further dry skin conditions. Itching symptoms may ease with antihistamine medication (Harding, 2016a).

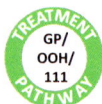

TREATMENT PATHWAY
GP/
OOH/
111

Intertrigo

Intertrigo (intertriginous dermatitis) is an inflammatory condition of skin folds affecting the axilla, perineum, breasts, abdominal folds, neck creases and sometimes between the fingers. It is generally caused by a lack of circulating air leading to increased heat, moisture or sweat and friction. It often becomes infected by Candida or bacterial mechanisms with patients suffering from chronic symptoms of itching and stinging within these skin folds (European Commission, 2016).

Symptoms

Intertrigo initially presents as erythematous (mild red) skin rash on both sides – a mirrored effect – of the skin folds which may progress to pustules, weeping lesions, erosions or fissures (PCDS, 2016c).

Monitor diabetic patients for infections

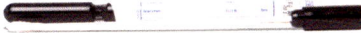

OTC

Emollients, barrier creams, talcum powders, antifungal creams

Treatment

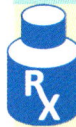

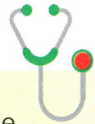

Check **BNF** dosage and local antimicrobial guidelines

✔ Topical treatment with antifungal creams such as **Clotrimizole 1%** which may be combined with a steroid cream) e.g. **trimovate**
✔ Topical or oral antibacterial treatment may also be indicated
✔ Antihistamine may relieve itching.

Patient advice includes:
■ General hygiene
■ Weight loss may be beneficial.

(PCDS, 2016c)

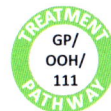

GP/ OOH/ 111

Nappy rash

A baby's skin is quite delicate and a nappy rash is a relatively common condition which is easily managed although the rash can become extremely sore very quickly. Preservatives found in some cleaning wipes such as methylisothiazolinone (MI) have been found to cause a variety of skin reactions too. European Union manufacturing legislation have now removed this from common products (CIRS, 2016).

Symptoms

Irritants in urine and faeces cause the skin to become inflamed leading to a hot red rash which can contain pimples and blisters.

Change the nappy regularly or leave the nappy off for long periods of time if possible. With each nappy change apply over-the-counter barrier preparations (NICE, 2018g):

✔ **Sudocrem**
✔ **Metanium**
✔ **Zinc and caster oils BP**
✔ **Paraffin BP ointments**
✔ **Bepanthen.**

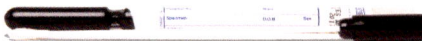

Treatment

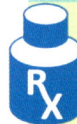

Check **BNF** dosage and local antimicrobial guidelines

Features may suggest a secondary infection. Fungal infections have sharp perimeter margins, treat with:
✔ **Clotrimazole 1% QDS**
✔ **Miconazole 2% BD**
✔ **Econazole 1% BD.**

Bacterial infections tend to have marked redness with exudate
✔ **Flucloxacillin**
✔ **Clarithromycin** if allergic to penicillin.

(NICE, 2018g)

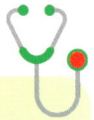

Hydrocortisone 1% ointment if severe. Do not use on open wounds.

TREATMENT GP/ OOH/ 111 PATHWAY

Skin swabs can be difficult to interpret as fungal and bacterial infections give similar results. Swab the area and send for laboratory analysis IF a secondary bacterial infection is suspected.

Fungal ear infection (Otomycosis)

Otomycosis is generally more common in hot climates and with people who swim a lot, take part in water sports or use hot tubs. It can also affect patients who wear hearing aids, use cotton buds or in-ear headphones although eczema can also trigger infections. History is very important!

Excessive swimming tends to have a washing effect to remove the cerumen (wax) which protects against many bacterial and fungal infections due to its acidic pH, therefore making the auditory canal more susceptible to fungal growth.

Symptoms

Clinical presentation is similar to bacterial otitis externa but fungal infections have long white fungal growths (filamentous hyphae) growing from the skin surface. Suspect a fungal infection if an infection does not respond to topical treatments such as Otomize®.

- ■ Clear the ear canal of debris and discharge several times a week
- ■ Keep the ear dry and avoid scratching it with cotton wool buds. Avoid cotton wool plugs in the ear unless discharge is profuse.

Treatment

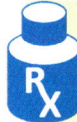

Check **BNF** dosage and local antimicrobial guidelines

Anti-fungal medications:
- ✔ **Analgesia** and **Burow's solution or 5% aluminium acetate solution** should be used to reduce the swelling and remove the debris
- ✔ Antifungal ear treatment **clotrimazole 1%** ear drops or **flumetasone pivalate 0.02% with clioquinol 1%**.

(NICE, 2018h)

Consider swab and send for fungal culture

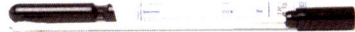

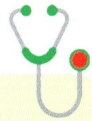

Antibiotic guidance for managing and treating common infections

Skin – fungal infections

Infection	Key points	Medicine	Adult doses	Length
Dermatophyte infection: skin	**Most cases**: terbinafine is fungicidal; treatment time shorter than fungistatic imidazoles. If candida possible, use imidazole.	Topical terbinafine OR Topical imidazole	1% OD–BD 1% OD–BD	1–4 wks 4–6 wks
	If intractable, or scalp: send skin scrapings. **If infection confirmed**: use oral terbinafine or itraconazole. **Scalp**: oral therapy, discuss with specialist.	For athlete's foot: topical undecenoates (e.g. Mycota®)	OD–BD	4–6 wks

Genital tract infections

Infection	Key points	Medicine	Adult doses	Length
STI screening	People with risk factors should be screened for chlamydia, gonorrhoea, HIV and syphilis. Refer individual and partners to GUM. Risk factors: <25 years; no condom use; recent/ frequent change of partner; symptomatic partner; area of high HIV.			
Chlamydia trachomatis/ urethritis	Opportunistically screen all patients aged 15–24 years annually and on change of sexual partner. If positive, treat index case, refer to GUM and initiate partner notification, testing and treatment. Advise patient with chlamydia to abstain from sexual intercourse until doxycycline is completed or for 7 days after treatment with azithromycin (14 days after azithromycin started and until symptoms resolved if urethritis).	First line: doxycycline	100 mg	7 days

	If chlamydia, test for reinfection at 3 to 6 months following treatment if under 25 years; or consider if over 25 years and high risk of re-infection.			
	Pregnancy/breastfeeding: azithromycin is most effective. As lower cure rate in pregnancy, test for cure at least three weeks after end of treatment.	azithromycin	1000 mg then 500 mg OD	Stat 2 days (total 3 days)
Epididymitis	Usually due to Gram-negative enteric bacteria in men over 35 years with low risk of STI. If under 35 years or STI risk, refer to GUM.	doxycycline	100 mg BD	10 to 14 days
		ofloxacin	200 mg BD	14 days
		ciprofloxacin	500 mg BD	10 days
Vaginal candidiasis	All topical and oral azoles give over 70% cure.	clotrimazole OR	500 mg pessary	Stat
	Pregnancy: avoid oral azoles and use intravaginal treatment for 7 days.	fenticonazole OR	600 mg pessary	Stat
		oral fluconazole OR	150 mg	Stat
		clotrimazole	100 mg pessary	6 nights
	Recurrent (>4 episodes per year): 150 mg oral fluconazole every 72 hours for three doses induction, followed by one dose once a week for six months maintenance.	Recurrent: Fluconazole (induction/ maintenance)	150 mg every 72 hours THEN 150 mg weekly	3 doses 6 months
Bacterial vaginosis	Oral metronidazole is as effective as topical treatment, and is cheaper. Seven days results in fewer relapses than 2 g stat at four weeks. **Pregnant/breastfeeding:** avoid 2 g dose. Treating partners does not reduce relapse.	Oral metronidazole OR	400 mg BD 2 g	7 days Stat
		metronidazole 0.75% vaginal gel OR	5 g app at night	5 nights
		clindamycin 2% cream	5 g app at night	7 nights

Oral candidiasis

Infection	Key points	Medicine	Adult doses	Length
Oral candidiasis	Topical azoles are more effective than topical nystatin. Oral candidiasis is rare in immunocompetent adults; consider undiagnosed risk factors, including HIV. Use 50 mg fluconazole if extensive/severe candidiasis; if HIV or immunocompromised, use 100 mg fluconazole.	Miconazole oral gel **If not tolerated:** Nystatin suspension Flucanozole capsules	2.5 ml of 24 mg/ml QDS (hold in mouth after food) 1 ml; 100,000 units/ ml QDS (half in each side) 50 mg/100 mg OD	7 days; continue for 7 days after resolved 7 days; continue for 2 days after resolved 7 to 14 days

Further Reading

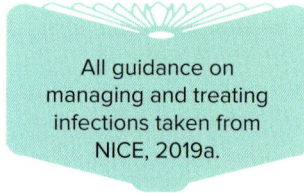

All guidance on managing and treating infections taken from NICE, 2019a.

Acne Vulgaris

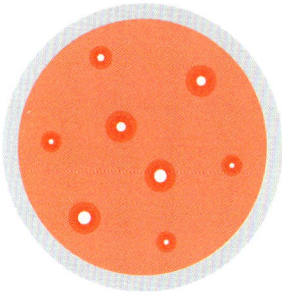

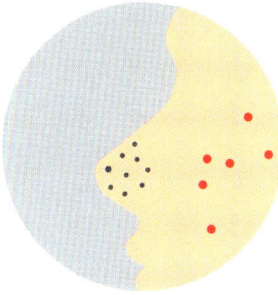

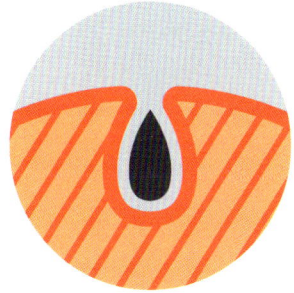

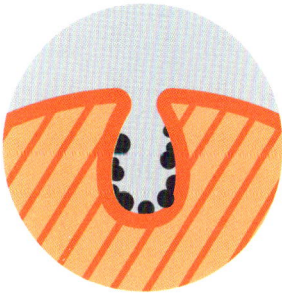

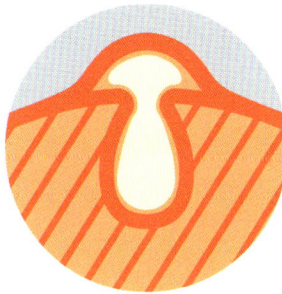

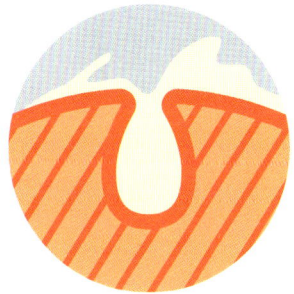

Key facts

Acne vulgaris is a chronic skin condition primarily occurring around puberty and affecting the majority of people at some point between 11 and 30 years of age (British Skin Foundation, 2019b; PCDS, 2019c; Dawson, 2013).

Acne is caused by a blockage or inflammation of the hair follicles and accompanying sebaceous glands so it mainly affects the face, back and chest areas. Mild or excessive eruptions can cause anxiety with younger adults as well as physical scarring or hyperpigmentation.

NICE recommended washing routines:

- Do not wash more than twice a day
- Use a mild soap or cleanser and lukewarm water
- Do not use vigorous scrubbing when washing acne-affected skin
- Do not use abrasive soaps, cleansing granules, astringents, or exfoliating agents
- Avoid excessive use of make-up and cosmetics
- Use a fragrance-free, water-based emollient if dry skin is a problem.

(NICE, 2018i)

- Treatment for acne can take up to 8 weeks to become effective and may also irritate the skin
- Topical and systemic antibiotics should not be prescribed together, or used as the sole treatment, as bacterial resistance is a growing concern
- All treatment should be routinely reviewed at 12 weeks
- In the event of pregnancy, topical retinoids and oral tetracyclines should be discontinued.

(NICE, 2018i)

Treatment

Benzoyl peroxide

Benzoyl peroxide is suitable for most people with acne of all severities, although it may irritate sensitive skin. It is available in a variety of strengths (2.5% to 10%) and formulations (cream, aqueous gel, gel and wash), available both on prescription and over the counter.

- Application is once or twice a day (once daily is usually sufficient) to all areas of the skin where acne occurs, not just active lesions
- Inform patients that topical treatments are effective and are worth persevering with. Improvements may not occur immediately and there may be an initial deterioration in the condition
- Areas that have been cleared of acne should also be treated until there is a likelihood the disease is in full remission (NICE, 2018i).

Topical retinoids

Topical retinoids have a preventative action against new lesions forming, as well as treating lesions that have already formed.

- They are contraindicated in pregnancy
- They can cause skin irritation, particularly in people with sensitive skin conditions such as eczema (NICE, 2018i).

A topical retinoid can be combined with a benzoyl peroxide for the maintenance of acne. Apply the products once daily, 12 hours apart (for example, the topical retinoid at night and benzoyl peroxide in the morning).

The drug should be applied sparingly — more is not better. A pea-sized amount of cream should be enough to treat the face.

Topical antibiotics

The topical antibiotic products that are licensed in the UK are:

- **Clindamycin** available as an aqueous solution, lotion, or gel (1%)
- **Erythromycin**, available as an alcoholic solution (2%) or gel (4%); or erythromycin (4%) combined with zinc (1.2%) in an alcoholic base.

Twice daily application, except for clindamycin gel which is licensed for once daily application. Topical antibiotics usually cause less irritation than benzoyl peroxide but where possible, treatment should be limited to 12 weeks duration (NICE, 2018i).

Oral antibiotics

Tetracyclines are considered first-line treatment if oral antibiotics are required. All are licensed for the treatment of acne vulgaris and there is no evidence that one is more effective than another. Therefore, the choice of specific tetracycline should be made according to the individual's preference and cost, bearing in mind the adverse affect profile of the drugs and the convenience of their dosing schedules.

- **Tetracycline** and **oxytetracycline** — the dose is 500 mg twice a day, on an empty stomach
- **Doxycycline** and **lymecycline** are taken once a day with food. Photosensitivity is reported to be a problem with doxycycline, so consider avoiding this in people who are exposed to a lot of sunlight
- **Minocycline** is not recommended for the treatment of acne.

Erythromycin is a suitable alternative to tetracycline if it is contraindicated (for example, in pregnancy). The dose is usually 500 mg twice a day (NICE, 2018i).

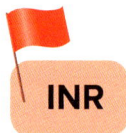

INR

Clindamycin can affect international normalised ratio (INR) tests and increase bleeding with the combined use of anticoagulants such as warfarin. INR tests should be more frequently monitored.

Azelaic acid

Azelaic acid is available as a cream and a gel:

- **Skinoren**® is a 20% cream licensed for acne vulgaris. It is applied twice a day, but this may be reduced to once a day during the first week if the person has sensitive skin. It is licensed for 6 months use, although it is frequently used for longer periods by specialists

- **Finacea**® is a 15% gel licensed for facial acne vulgaris. It is applied twice a day and can be continued over several months according to clinical outcome, although it should be stopped after 1 month if there is no improvement or deterioration occurs.

Azelaic acid causes less skin irritation than topical retinoid or benzoyl peroxide but can lighten the colour of the skin. It is a second-line option that should be considered if other treatments are unsuitable (NICE, 2018i).

Combined oral contraceptives

Treatment with a combined oral contraceptive (COC) should be considered for all women with acne who require contraception or in whom there is a suspected hormonal basis for the acne (NICE, 2018i).

Further Reading

Information on treating acne vulgaris taken from NICE, 2018i.

The prescribing of COC needs to be discussed with the patient's GP or specialised clinician.

Treatment for acne is considered in three main stages of severity.
MILD – MODERATE – SEVERE

Mild acne

Mild acne consists of open and closed comedones (black-/whiteheads) and a single topical treatment should be prescribed:

- Topical retinoid (tretinoin, isotretinoin, or adapalene) or benzoyl peroxide (especially if papules and pustules are present) as first-line treatment
- Azelaic acid should be prescribed if both topical retinoids and benzoyl peroxide are poorly tolerated
- Prescription of a standard combined oral contraceptive should be considered in women who require contraception.

Moderate acne

Moderate acne consists of papules and pustules (inflammatory lesions), which may be widespread with a risk of scarring and psychological issues.

- A single topical drug should be considered for people with limited acne which is unlikely to scar (benzoyl peroxide or a topical retinoid)
- Combined treatment should be considered for all people with moderate acne. A topical antibiotic combined with benzoyl peroxide or a topical retinoid is the preferred regimen, as it is proven to be effective and may limit the development of bacterial resistance. Where possible, a topical antibiotic course should be limited to a maximum of 12 weeks
- An oral antibiotic (tetracyclines or erythromycin) combined with a topical treatment (but not a topical antibiotic) should be considered if there is moderate acne on the back or shoulders, or if there is a significant risk of scarring or substantial pigment change. A standard combined oral contraceptive should be considered in women who require contraception.

Severe acne

Severe acne consists of nodules and cysts as well as inflammatory papules and pustules. There is a high risk of scarring and there is likely to be considerable psychosocial morbidity.

- All people with severe acne should be referred for specialist assessment and treatment

- Prescription of an oral antibiotic in combination with a topical drug should be considered while waiting for an appointment. Prescription of a combined oral contraceptive (COC) should be considered for women who require contraception. Standard COCs are suitable for most women.

- Co-cyprindiol (Dianette®) should be considered only when topical treatment or systemic antibiotics have failed.

Further Reading

For more details on treatment pathways for acne see Bewley, 2015.

Evaluation of Melanoma and Pigmented Lesions

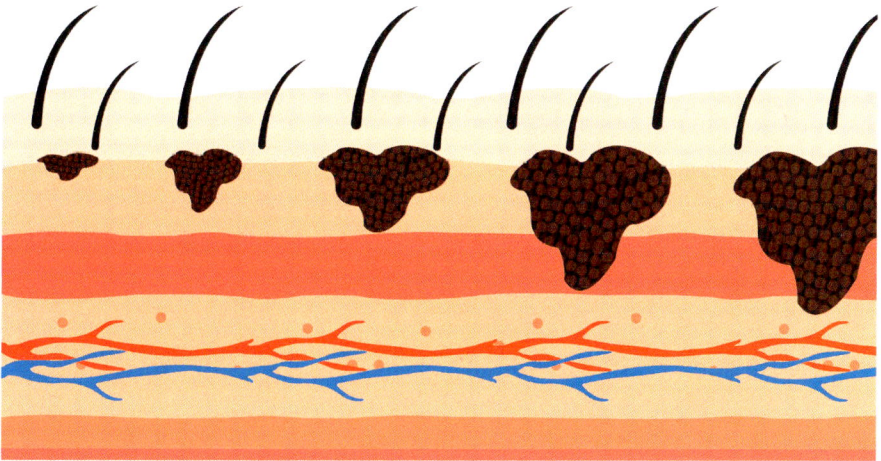

Skin cancer variations

Cancer Research UK (2017) distinguish between two main types of skin cancer:

- Non-melanoma
- Melanoma

Non-melanoma

Non-melanoma skin cancer is different from melanoma and includes two main types:

- Basal cell skin cancer (BCC)
- Squamous cell skin cancer (SCC)

The variants are named after the types of skin cells where the cancer develops although it is possible for a non-melanoma skin cancer to be a mixture of both BCC and SCC.

Basal cell cancers usually develop on areas exposed to the sun, especially the face, head and neck, but they can occur anywhere on the body. The cancers are often fragile and might bleed after shaving or after a minor injury, taking a long time to heal.

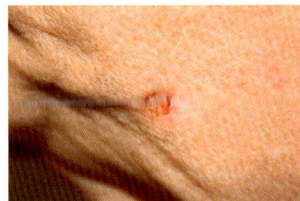

BCC is rarely fatal but if it is not diagnosed early enough, or treated properly it can result in tumours that disfigure or even destroy important anatomical structures such as the nose, eyes, ears and lips. This can make it a more challenging condition to treat if the tumour becomes inoperable.

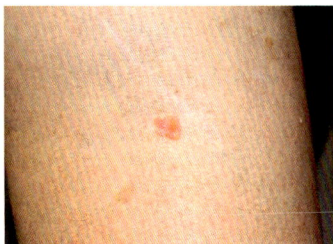

Squamous cell cancers also develop on sun-exposed areas of the body but less often in the genital area.

SCC can be disfiguring and can be fatal if it spreads. Its development is associated with chronic ultraviolet radiation exposure in the earlier decades of life (Leiter et al., 2008).

Basal cell cancers

Symptoms

Appearance can vary. Look for areas of the skin that are either:

- Flat, firm, pale or yellow, similar to a scar
- Raised reddish patches that might be itchy
- Small, pink or red, translucent, shiny, pearly bumps, which might have blue, brown or black areas
- Pink growths with raised edges and a lower area in their centre, which might contain abnormal blood vessels in a spreading formation.

Look for open sores which may have oozing or crusted areas that do not heal, or recurrent sores in the same places.

Squamous cell cancers

Symptoms

Appearance can vary. Look for areas of the skin that are either:

- Rough or scaly red patches, which might crust or bleed
- Raised growths or lumps, sometimes with a lower area in the centre
- Open sores (which may have oozing or crusted areas) that don't heal, or that heal and then come back
- Wart-like growths.

Both basal and squamous cell skin cancers can also develop as a flat area showing only slight changes from normal skin.

Melanoma

Melanoma, also known as malignant melanoma, is a type of skin cancer caused by the abnormal proliferation of melanocytes containing pigment (see page 19). Most pigment cells are found in the skin with certain areas being more prone to proliferation than others. In men, the areas most likely to be affected are the chest and the back, but in women, the legs are the most common site (NCRAS, 2012). Other common sites are the neck and face; melanoma can also occur in the eyes and is known as ocular melanoma. Melanoma is just one type of skin cancer and is less common than basal cell or squamous cell skin cancers, but it can be dangerous as it is more likely to become metastatic.

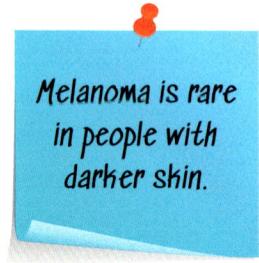

Melanoma is rare in people with darker skin.

It is worth considering that the earlier the diagnosis the lower the metastatic risk. The main aim of prevention campaigns and clinicians working in primary care is to improve the early diagnosis of melanoma risks. The curability of skin cancer is very high if it is recognised early enough and treated surgically (Alender, 2009).

Melanoma is described as:

- **In situ** – if confined to the epidermis
- **Invasive** – if spread to the dermis
- **Metastatic** – if spread to other tissues from the skin.

(Oakley, 2015).

Malignant melanoma is the most serious skin cancer and is responsible for the majority of skin cancer deaths. Treatment is more likely to be successful when it is caught early. It has consistently been associated with intermittent sun exposure mostly accrued through recreational activities (Gallagher, 2006; Gandini, 2005; Walter, 1999).

Melanoma is the type of skin cancer that most often develops from a mole. This can be a mole that is already on the skin or one that has recently appeared. The appearance of a malignant melanoma depends on its type and site.

There are four common subtypes of melanoma:

- Superficial spreading melanoma
- Nodular melanoma
- Lentigo maligna melanoma
- Acral lentiginous melanoma

Superficial spreading melanoma, nodular melanoma and lentigo maligna melanoma make up 90% of all diagnosed malignant melanomas, with acral lentiginous melanoma and a few very rare types making up the other 10% (NHS, 2017b).

Superficial spreading melanoma

Superficial spreading melanoma is the most common type of melanoma. It often remains in situ for long periods and usually spreads horizontally. This characteristic growth is known as having a 'radial growth phase'. Superficial spreading melanoma may present as a flat, pigmented lesion with asymmetrical or irregular borders. It is usually identified in the fourth to fifth decades and most commonly found on sun-exposed sites.

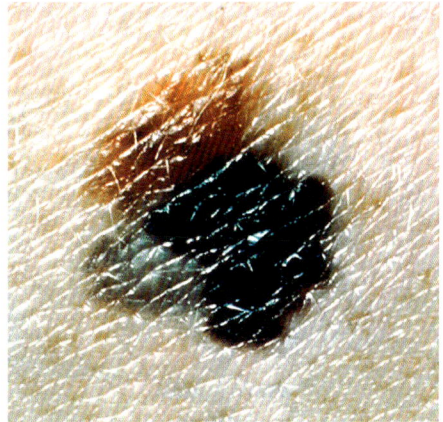

Nodular melanoma

Nodular melanoma is the second most common subtype of melanoma and often presents as an atypical nodule that may ulcerate and bleed easily. It may be difficult to diagnose as it can present as a darkly pigmented lesion or red/pink in colour. It usually presents from the fifth or sixth decade and commonly occurs on the legs or trunk. Nodular melanoma has a vertical growth pattern and thus can spread rapidly in comparison to other forms of melanoma (Kalkhoran, 2010).

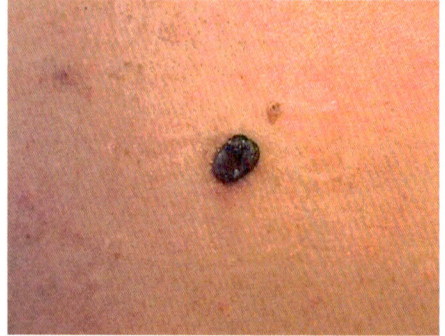

Lentigo maligna

Lentigo maligna is also known as Hutchinson's melanotic freckle and is a precursor to lentigo maligna melanoma. The cancerous cells of lentigo maligna are in situ and present as a slow-growing patch of brown skin, often resembling a freckle in its early stages (PCDS, 2017b). Lesions take several years to grow and are most common in older people on sun-exposed skin, most often found on the head and neck (BAD, 2014).

Lentigo maligna melanoma

Lentigo maligna melanoma develops from a preinvasive phase lentigo maligna (PCDS, 2017). It is an irregularly shaped brown macule which grows slowly, and over time may develop irregular colours (dark brown, black, blue). Lentigo maligna melanoma usually grows horizontally initially but can form nodules once it enters the vertical growth phase.

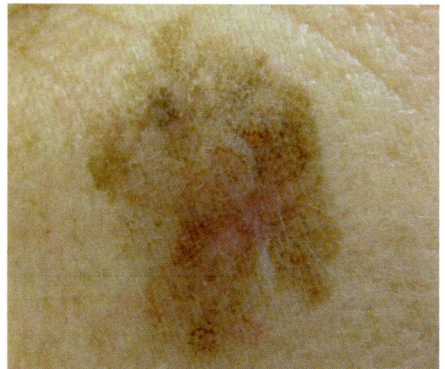

Acral lentiginous melanoma

Acral lentiginous melanoma is more common on the soles of the feet but can be found on the palms of hands or the nail bed. It presents with a flat, pigmented area slowly increasing in size, becoming increasingly irregular in colour and border. It may be covered with reactive callus if on the sole and eventually may develop a nodule with ulceration and bleeding. There may be brown or black discolouration (Hutchinson's sign) in advanced growth. It can occur in all ethnic groups but is most common in darker skin types (Oakley, 2015).

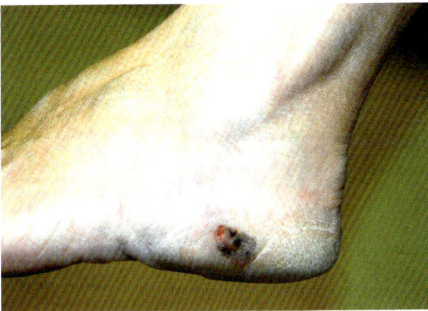

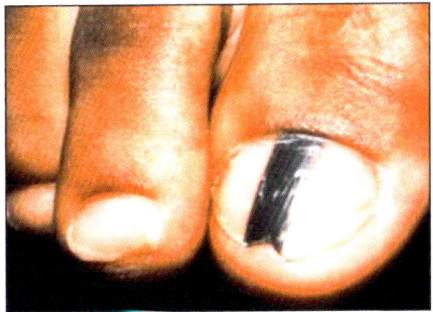

Risk factors

Some of the known factors that increase the risk of melanoma include:

- A personal or family history of skin cancer
- Pale skin (Fitzpatrick Skin Type I and II) that burns easily
- Red, blonde or light-coloured hair
- Blue or green eyes
- History of sunburn, particularly blistering sunburn in childhood
- A large number of moles
- Unusually high sun exposure – especially those who mainly work outside
- Use of tanning beds or sun beds
- Increasing age – the incidence of malignant melanoma increases with age in both men and women, from 15 years of age onwards.

Recommended preventative advice

- **Wear sunscreen**. UV radiation can still damage skin in the winter so use a broad-spectrum sunscreen daily with a protective factor of at least 30. In a 2003 survey, 80% of those questioned mentioned using sunscreen to reduce the risk of skin cancer, but less than 44% specifically mentioned using a sunscreen with a 15+ SPF (Office for National Statistics, 2003)
- **Wear protective clothing**. Wear sun-protective clothing, hat, and sunglasses
- **Avoid peak rays**. Midday sun rays are most intense
- **Avoid use of tanning beds**. Indoor tanning has been shown to increase the risk of melanoma by up to 75%.

Further Reading

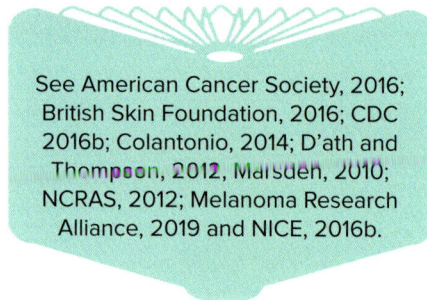

See American Cancer Society, 2016; British Skin Foundation, 2016; CDC 2016b; Colantonio, 2014; D'ath and Thompson, 2012, Marsden, 2010; NCRAS, 2012; Melanoma Research Alliance, 2019 and NICE, 2016b.

Diagnosis

Diagnostic tools

In primary care settings, distinguishing melanomas from other pigmented skin lesions can be very challenging. There are two main scoring systems used which aid clinicians with visual inspection of a pigmented skin lesion and help identify those that require urgent referral for suspected melanoma.

- The weighted 7-point checklist (formally just 7-point) checklist
- ABCDE checklist.

Although both of these systems are fairly similar and widely used, the weighted 7-point checklist has been recommended by NICE (2017g) for routine use in UK general practice to identify clinically significant lesions which require urgent referral. Some clinicians may be more familiar with, or even still practise, the ABCDE system so it has been included for reference.

Further Reading

Further reading for both diagnostic systems includes Healsmith, 1994; NICE, 2017f; Walker, 2013.

Weighted 7-point checklist

The 7-point checklist (7PCL) was developed in Glasgow circa 1980 as guidance for GPs and patients to detect a possible melanoma. Each feature will score 1 and lesions with scores of more than 3 would be referred to dermatology for further assessment.

The 7PCL was then revised in 1989 and is now called the weighted 7-point checklist and used to identify three major signs:

- Change in size
- Change in shape
- Change in colour.

And four minor signs:

- Inflammation
- Crusting or bleeding
- Sensory changes
- A diameter greater than 7 mm.

For a suspected malignant melanoma the scoring is weighted, meaning that each major sign now scores 2 and minor signs score 1. Any lesion scoring more than 3 will be referred to dermatology.

Symptoms

Major features (2 points)
- Change in size of lesion
- Irregular pigmentation
- Irregular border.

Minor features (1 point)
- Inflammation
- Itch or altered sensation
- Larger than other lesions (diameter >7 mm)
- Oozing/crusting of lesion.

Refer patients for a suspected melanoma using a cancer pathway ensuring an appointment within 2 weeks IF they have a suspicious pigmented skin lesion with a weighted 7-point checklist score of 3 or more.

ABCDE checklist

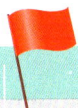

Asymmetry

An unremarkable mole is generally symmetrical and grows relatively evenly. If you divided the mole in half then each side would be a mirror image of the other

A suspect lesion would be asymmetrical and the two halves would differ in shape

Border

Normal moles tend to be much rounder, with smooth, clearly defined borders

Melanomas often have irregular, blurred borders or edges

Colour

Normal lesions have one uniform colour

Melanomas are often uneven in colour and can have different shades of brown or black, or varying shades of red and pink.

The darkening of a mole is a sign that it is possibly becoming cancerous

Diameter

Normal lesions are usually less than 6 mm in diameter

Most melanomas are larger than 6 mm in diameter

Enlargement

The original mole often remains the same size

A melanoma will change in size becoming raised above the skin's surface. Inflammation, swelling bleeding, itching or crusting may also be melanoma red flags

Stage scoring systems

The stage at which a cancer is diagnosed will indicate how far it has already spread and what kind of treatment is suitable. There are several variations of stage scoring systems used (Cancer Research UK, 2015).

> There are two scales, the Clark scale and the Breslow scale, which describe how deep the melanoma is within the skin.

The Clark scale

The Clark scale is a way of measuring how deeply the melanoma has grown into the skin and which levels of the skin are affected. It has five levels:

- **Level 1** – also called melanoma in situ as the melanoma cells are in the epidermis only
- **Level 2** – melanoma cells now within the papillary dermis
- **Level 3** – melanoma cells have spread throughout the papillary dermis and have now breached the reticular dermis
- **Level 4** – melanoma has spread into the reticular or deep dermis
- **Level 5** – melanoma has grown into the subcutaneous fat layer.

The Breslow scale

The Breslow scale is used by the pathologist to measures the thickness of the melanoma with a micrometer. This will indicate how far the melanoma cells have progressed through the skin layers from the epidermis. The Breslow thickness is used in the TNM staging system for melanoma.

> **TNM stands for Tumour, Node, Metastasis**

The TNM system

The TNM system describes the size of the initial cancer or primary tumour and whether the cancer has spread to the lymph nodes or metastasised. The system uses letters and numbers to describe the cancer:

T – refers to the size of the cancer and how far it has spread into nearby tissue – it can be 1, 2, 3 or 4, with 1 being small and 4 large

N – refers to whether the cancer has spread to the lymph nodes – it can be between 0 meaning no lymph nodes contain cancer cells and 3 meaning multiple lymph nodes contain cancer cells

M – refers to whether the cancer has metastasised. It can either be 0 meaning the cancer hasn't spread, or 1 meaning the cancer has spread.

So in summary, the grading looks at the melanoma depth, and also whether the melanoma has spread to the lymph nodes or to another part of the body. The classification given to a cancer by the TNM system is used in the numbered staging system to identify the stage of the cancer.

Numbered staging system

- **Stage 0:** The cancer is only in the outermost layer of skin and is described as melanoma in situ
- **Stage 1:** The cancer is up to 2 mm thick. It has not spread to the lymph nodes or any other sites and ulceration may or may not be evident
- **Stage 2:** The cancer is at least 1.01 mm thick and it may be thicker than 4 mm. It has not spread to the lymph nodes or any other sites and ulceration may or may not be evident
- **Stage 3:** The cancer has spread to one or more of the lymph nodes or nearby lymphatic channels, but not to distant sites.The original cancer may no longer be visible. If it is visible, it may be thicker than 4 mm, and it may also be ulcerated
- **Stage 4:** The cancer has spread to distant lymph nodes or organs, such as the brain, lungs or liver.

Differential diagnosis

The key question to ask is could the lesion could be a malignant melanoma? SEEK ADVICE!

Further Reading

For more information see Cancer Research UK, 2019.

Although there are several characteristic features of melanoma, it can be difficult to differentiate melanoma from other lesions. Not all changes in the skin are a sign of cancer. Below are some common examples.

Actinic keratoses, also known as solar keratoses, are dry, scaly patches of skin caused by damage from years of sun exposure. The patches can be pink, red or brown, and can vary in size from a few millimetres to a few centimetres across. The affected skin can sometimes become very thick, and occasionally the patches can look like small horns or spikes. There's a small risk that the patches could develop into squamous cell carcinoma if untreated. See also pages 128–129 for more detail on actinic keratosis

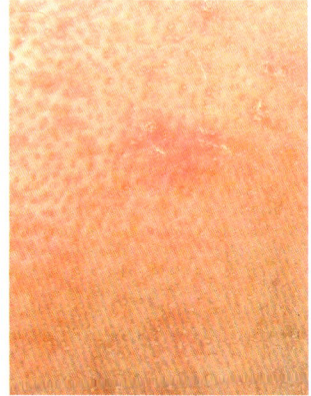

Seborrhoeic keratoses (SK) are also known as seborrhoeic warts or basal cell papillomas. They are benign growths due to a build-up of skin cells which are very common, harmless, often pigmented, growths on the skin.

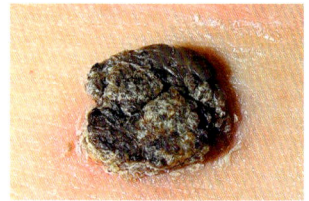

Dermatofibromas are firm lumps usually less than 1 cm in diameter and range from pink to brown in colour, often in a ring around the fibrous knot of tissue. Most commonly they occur on the lower legs of young or middle-aged adults and are more common in women than men.

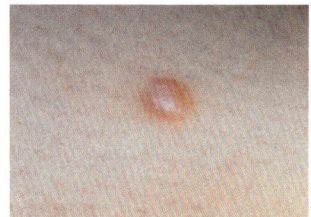

Referral

Melanoma

Refer people using a suspected cancer pathway referral (for an appointment within 2 weeks) if dermoscopy suggests melanoma of the skin.

Consider a suspected cancer pathway referral (for an appointment within 2 weeks) for melanoma in people with a pigmented or non-pigmented skin lesion that suggests nodular melanoma.

Squamous cell carcinoma

Consider a suspected cancer pathway referral (for an appointment within 2 weeks) for people with a skin lesion that raises the suspicion of squamous cell carcinoma.

Basal cell carcinoma

Consider routine referral for people if they have a skin lesion that raises the suspicion of a basal cell carcinoma. NICE have now suggested that a possible basal cell carcinoma may warrant a 2-week referral but to only consider a suspected cancer pathway referral (for an appointment within 2 weeks) for people with a skin lesion for which there is particular concern that a delay may have a significant impact, because of factors such as lesion site or size (NICE, 2019g).

Common Skin Conditions in Primary Care

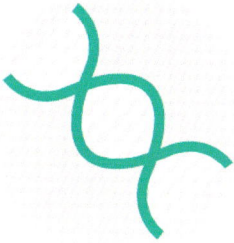

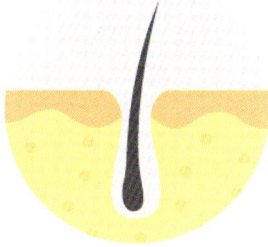

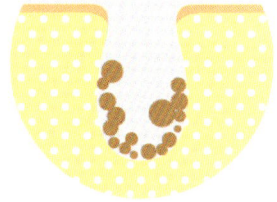

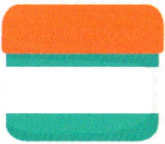

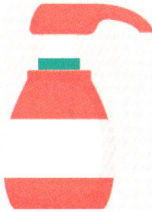

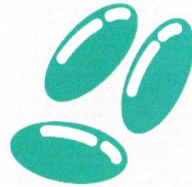

Actinic keratosis

Actinic keratosis is also known as solar keratosis. 'Actinic' and 'solar' mean 'sunlight-induced' in Greek and Latin, respectively. Keratosis refers to thickened skin. Patients taking immunosuppressive drugs or who have actinic keratosis are more at risk of all types of skin cancer compared to someone of the same age without actinic keratosis (BAD, 2016).

The condition is not contagious and is caused by long-term exposure to the sun and is therefore more common in older generations. It can also affect pale skinned, red haired or blonde people who burn easily in the sun.

Symptoms

The lesions are usually formed in areas which have high exposure to the sun such as the forearms, dorsum of hands, the face, ears and bald patches on the top of heads.

Lump becomes tender

Sores that bleed or don't heal

Treatment

Treatments used for actinic keratoses include the following:

✔ Freezing with liquid nitrogen (cryotherapy)
✔ Surgical removal is another option, but the risk of scarring is high. A skin sample can be analysed in the laboratory to confirm a diagnosis.
✔ Topical creams can be prescribed and may include 5-fluorouracil, imiquimod or ingenol mebutate gel although these tend to cause inflammation. Diclofenac and retinoic acid are alternatives to consider as they cause milder side effects.
✔ Laser treatment may be useful, particularly for actinic keratosis on the lips.

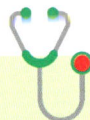

(BAD, 2016)

Protecting skin from the sun with sunscreen of factor 30 or more and wearing hats, long sleeves etc. will help reduce further actinic keratoses and also reduce the risk of getting a sun-induced skin cancer. Patients should avoid artificial sunlamps, including sunbeds and UV tanning cabinets too. Advise patients that if an actinic keratosis shows signs of change such as swelling, bleeding, itching or pus exudate then review with a GP or suitable clinician.

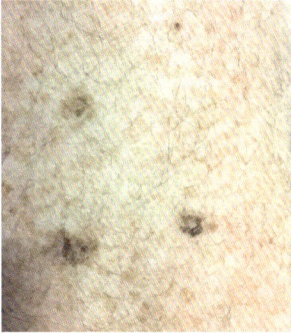

Actinic keratosis can be very diverse in appearance, presenting singularly or in clusters so can easily confuse diagnosis.

They may grow up to a centimetre or more in size and can occasionally develop into a thick, scaly layer similar to a wart with the surrounding skin looking sun damaged, blotchy, freckled or wrinkled.

If an actinic keratosis develops these symptoms then medical advice should be sought as this could indicate the early onset of a squamous cell carcinoma (cancer).

Further Reading

See BAD, 2016 for more information on actinic keratosis.

Boils and carbuncles

Most boils are caused by a Staphylococcus aureus bacteria which enters the body through lesions in the skin or via the hair follicles. The most common places for boils to appear are on the face, neck, armpits, shoulders and buttocks. If several boils appear in a group or within very close proximity of each other then this is called a carbuncle, which is generally a more serious type of infection (PCDS, 2018a).

Most boils burst and heal by themselves without causing any further problems although some patients may develop a deeper secondary infection such as cellulitis or even sepsis. Larger boils and carbuncles can also cause scarring.

Symptoms

- Initially the skin turns red around the infection
- A tender lump develops
- At 4 to 7 days, the lump starts turning white as pus collects under the skin
- May feel unwell and have pyrexia.

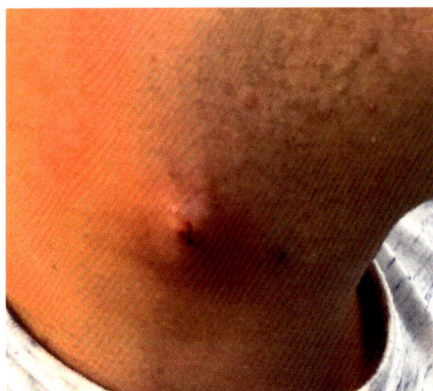

Treatment

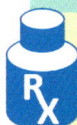

Check **BNF** dosage and local antimicrobial guidelines

Consider antibiotics:

✔ **Flucloxacillin** or **Co-amoxiclav**

✔ **Clarithromycin.**

Consider the needs/benefits of incising and drainage.

Discuss with duty doctor for clarification or referral to hospital.

Apply a warm compress for 10–20 minutes 3 or 4 times a day.

(NICE, 2017g)

TREATMENT PATHWAY
GP/ OOH/ 111

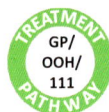

Carbuncle requires review

Cellulitis and erysipelas

Symptoms

Erysipelas is a superficial dermal infection which mainly affects the upper dermal layers only and is typically raised and demarcated.

Cellulitis is a deeper infection of the dermis which is also affecting the subcutaneous tissues. This can be difficult for clinicians to differentiate and diagnosis is usually a judgement of how serious the presenting symptoms are. An infection will have signs of tracking with well demarcated edges, which can be swollen and hot to touch.

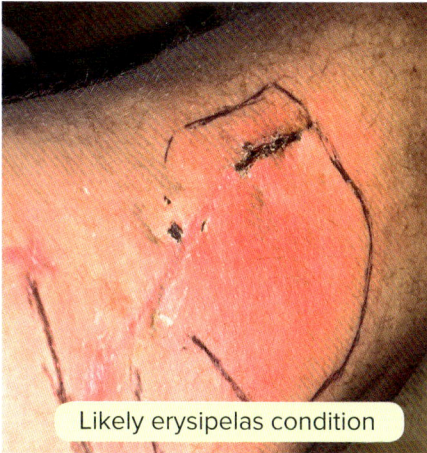

Likely erysipelas condition

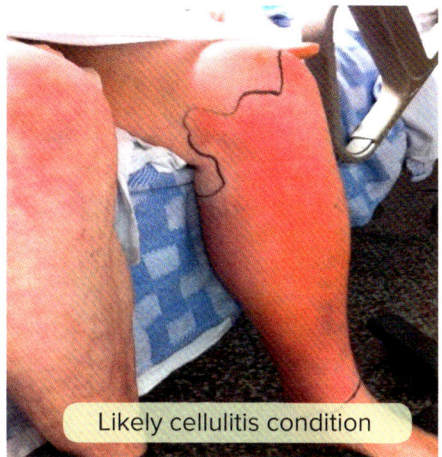

Likely cellulitis condition

Points to consider for diagnosis

- A common cause of cellulitis is athlete's foot
- Other causes are small local lesions or eczema
- Cellulitis commonly affects lower limbs
- Similar signs and levels of redness or infection in both legs is unlikely to be cellulitis. It is highly unlikely that a bacteria has entered at exactly the same point and time then progressed simultaneously on each leg at the same rate (Higuera, 2019).

Cellulitis can be divided into different classes of infection depending on the clinical presentation and history:

- **Class I** – afebrile and generally well/mild symptoms systemically
- **Class II** – febrile and unwell
- **Class III** – toxic appearance.

(NICE, 2019h)

Treatment

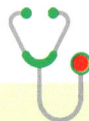

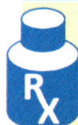

Check **BNF** dosage and local antimicrobial guidelines

Class I

✔ **Flucloxacillin QDS** 10 days.

If mildly systemically unwell
✔ **Flucloxacillin QDS** and **amoxicillin TDS.**

If penicillin allergy then
✔ **Clarithromycin** 10 days.

If patient is on statins then consider
✔ **Doxycycline** 200 mg initially then 100 mg daily 10 days.

(NICE, 2019h)

Class II and Class III Cellulitis (NICE, 2019h)

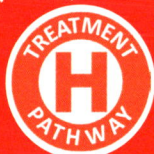

TREATMENT
H
PATHWAY

May require IV antibiotics and admission to hospital

TREATMENT
GP/
OOH/
111
PATHWAY

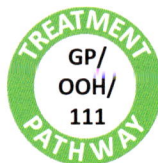

Other risk factors to consider are diabetes, immunosuppressed patients and drug addicts.

Comedones (blackheads)

During puberty, oil production in the sebaceous glands increases which can lead to comedones or blackheads as well as acne, although acne is also found in premenstrual women with polycystic ovarian syndrome.

The pilosebaceous unit is a collection of dermal structures consisting of:

■ Hair and the hair follicle
■ Arrector pili muscles
■ Sebaceous glands.

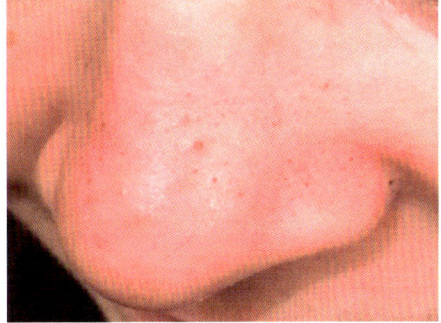

Symptoms

Comedones are associated with the pilosebaceous unit which are found in large quantities around the face, neck, upper chest, shoulders and back. The hair follicle can easily become blocked by excess keratin and sebum production and is called a microcomedo. If sebum continues to build up behind this blockage it can form a visible comedo (Williams, 2012).

Treatment

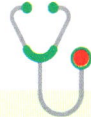

A topical retinoid is needed as this reduces comedones activity. Although topical retinoids should be avoided in pregnancy, they are safe to use in all other patients including sexually active women. Prescription options include:

✔ Adapalene (Differin®)

✔ Adapalene combined with benzoyl peroxide 2.5% (Epiduo®)

✔ Isotretinoin (e.g. Isotrex®)

✔ Azelaic acid.

(NHS, 2019b)

A comedo may be open to the environmental air which causes an oxidation process turning the area black (blackhead) whereas a closed area not affected by the environmental air remains white (whitehead). Solar comedones (sometimes called senile comedones) are related to several years of exposure to the sun and are not acne-related.

- Having blackheads is not an indication of dirty or unclean skin
- Washing or scrubbing the skin too much could make it worse
- Make-up and skin products that are oil-free and water-based may be less likely to cause acne and comedones
- A hair that does not emerge normally can also block the pore and cause a bulge or lead to infection.

Folliculitis

Folliculitis is a common skin condition seen within primary care clinics and although the condition isn't serious, it can become extremely sore or itchy (pruritus) for the patient with more severe infections possibly leading to hair loss and scarring.

Hair follicles can become inflamed or infected by:

- **Bacteria**, usually Staphylococcus aureus which resides on the skin surface
- **Fungal** infections which are generally associated with hot tubs and pools
- **Gram-negative** folliculitis can affect patients who are taking long-term medications for conditions such as eczema
- **Tinea barbae** is another fungal (dermatophyte) infection found commonly in men who shave against the hair follicle growth
- **Herpetic folliculitis** is due to the herpes simplex virus (HSV) and is often found in men who shave near oral cold sore lesions.

Symptoms

- Small red bumps or white-headed pimples around hair follicles
- Itchy, burning, tender skin
- The infection can also spread and develop into non-healing crusty sores or a large swollen mass.

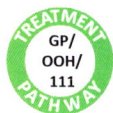

Mild or superficial folliculitis may resolve without treatment.

Treatment

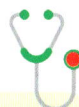

Check **BNF** dosage and local antimicrobial guidelines

✔ Pharmacological treatment is dependent on the type of infection:

Nasal (S. aureus)
✔ Topical Fucidin®

Bacterial folliculitis
✔ Flucloxacillin or clarithromycin

Pseudomonas folliculitis
✔ Oral ciprofloxacin

Fungal infections
✔ Clotrimazole or oral ketoconazole

Herpetic folliculitis
✔ Aciclovir or similar.

(Knott, 2017)

Hand, foot and mouth disease

Nothing to do with sheep! It is usually a mild infection caused by the Coxsackie A16 virus or similar viral groups. It is a self-limiting condition without the need for antibiotics.

Symptoms

- Crops of small spots (vesicles) appear around the mouth, hands and feet
- Child may sometimes present unwell; it will be due to a secondary infection such as a respiratory tract infection rather than HFM in isolation
- Child may also complain of a sore throat and lethargy.

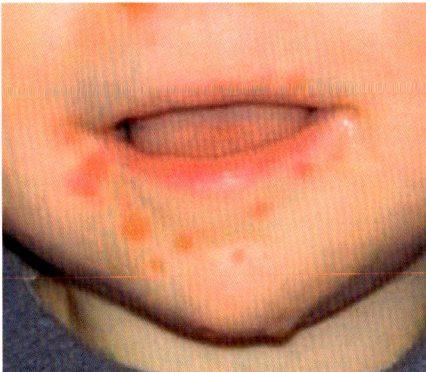

Treatment

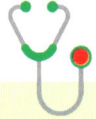

- Maintain fluids/ hydration
- Soothing mouth washes
- Avoid fruits/juices as this may cause pain from the mouth ulcers
- Average duration 7 days
- Monitor for secondary infections
- Ensure good hand hygiene.

(NHS Inform, 2019b)

OTC Manage pyrexia with paracetamol and ibuprofen

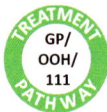

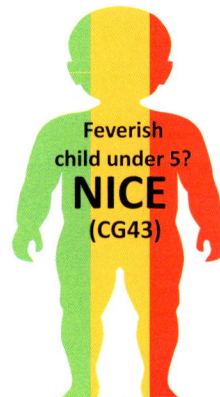

Feverish child under 5?
NICE (CG43)

TREATMENT GP/ OOH/ 111 PATHWAY

Head lice

Infestation from the head lice parasite (Pediculus humanus capitis) is a very common condition affecting all ages of patient. This type of parasite is only specific to humans and it feeds on blood while living its complete life cycle on the human scalp. It is specific to the scalp while different type of species infest other body areas.

Female lice live for up to 40 days and can lay 100+ eggs which they attach to hairs close to the scalp surface. The eggs are very small and usually yellow or white in colour, taking 7 to 10 days to hatch. It only takes a further 7 days before the new lice are able to lay their own eggs making them a troublesome and resilient problem to cure (BAD, 2017b).

Contrary to certain myths, head lice cannot fly, jump or burrow into the scalp, they live in long or short hair and pass over by close contact with other people who are infected.
Dirty hair is NOT a main contributing factor.

Symptoms

- Itching due to a reaction to the saliva of lice is usually a telltale sign
- Finding live lice/eggs.

Wet combing must be actioned for at least 2 weeks regularly to be successful, or continued until no lice have been seen for 3+ combing sessions (NHS, 2018f).

Nits are the empty egg cases attached to hair.

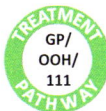

Treatment

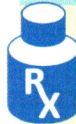

Check **BNF** dosage and **over-the-counter remedies**

✔ **Dimeticone** 4%: lotion, spray, gel – suitable for children 6 months+. Use regularly until infestation is controlled (NICE, 2016c).

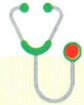

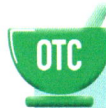

GP/ OOH/ 111

TREATMENT PATHWAY

OTC Other products including specific insecticides are also available.

Heat rash (prickly heat)

Anyone can develop a prickly heat rash. Major contributing factors are being in a hot climate or in situations where you sweat more than usual. Clothing can also exacerbate symptoms because of the sweating, heat and friction of the clothes on the skin leading to irritation. Higher risk groups include those with immobility or obesity.

Symptoms

The condition is caused when the body's sweat glands become blocked causing fluid to become trapped under the superficial dermal layers. This initially presents as small, clear blisters leading to formation of itchy red bumps (papules).

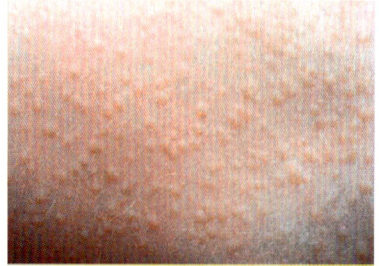

Compared to adults, infants have reduced ability to sweat because of the immaturity of their eccrine (sweat) glands therefore they are more prone to overheating. This presents as itchy red bumps (papules) known as **miliaria rubra** but is still a prickly heat rash (NHS, 2018g).

Parents may also report a history of a varying severity regarding the rash, especially at bath time, so bear in mind that this may have looked much worse prior to them coming in for a clinical consultation. The history can actually work in our favour as clinicians and we can use this example as reassurance to the parents that the rash is heat-related and the variations are due to babies' inability to moderate temperature.

OTC
- ✔ **Calamine lotion**
- ✔ **Low-strength hydrocortisone cream. Not to the face.**
- ✔ **Antihistamine medication.**

Treatment

- Avoid excessive heat and humidity
- Avoid tight synthetic fibres, such as polyester and nylon
- Drink plenty of fluids
- Apply cold compress no longer than 20 minutes.

(NHS, 2018e)

Henoch-Schönlein purpura

Henoch-Schönlein purpura (HSP) is not a common condition but mainly affects children under the age of 10 years old (NHS Foundation Trust, 2019).

HSP can resolve without complications although some patients may be at risk of renal failure. Normal recovery is around 4 weeks although the hospital may request regular blood pressure checks and urinalysis post-referral if HSP is diagnosed.

Symptoms

A non-blanching rash is caused by inflammation of the blood vessels (vasculitis) initiated by an abnormal immune system response. A pinpoint rash is described as **petechial** while larger rashes are described as **purpuric**.

■ Abdominal pains

■ Aching joints

■ May have been preceded by a primary infection such as a common cold with pyrexia.

Treatment

■ Most cases will be managed in secondary care. In primary care, provide a rapid assessment and then refer (PCDS, 2019d).

■ Monitor blood pressure

■ Has a recent medication caused these symptoms? If yes then stop.

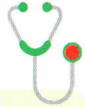

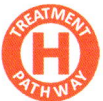

Consider meningitis!

Further Reading

For more details see Salama, 2016.

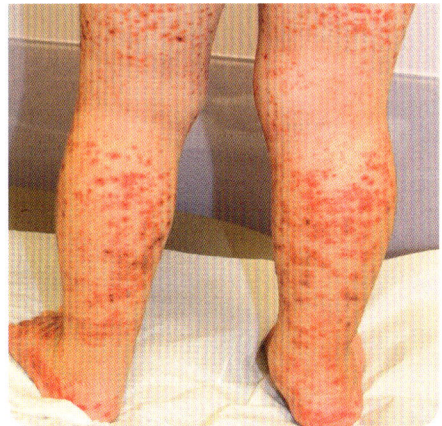

Herpes

The herpes simplex virus remains in the body for life but stays inactive most of the time. On occasions the virus is reactivated causing new symptoms to present, although these tend to be of a milder intensity than the initial outbreak. Signs of infection present within around 4 to 7 days after exposure, but sometimes it can be months or even years after getting infected before symptoms first appear.

Contamination is through skin-to-skin contact usually during vaginal, oral or anal sexual activity as the virus can enter the body through the moist skin of the mouth, penis, vagina and rectum.

There are two types of herpes simplex, **HSV-1** and **HSV-2**, and both types can cause:

- Cold sores on the mouth
- Genital herpes
- Whitlows on the fingers and hands (THT, 2019).

There are eight currently identified members of the herpes virus family:

- **Herpes simplex type I** (HSV-1)
- **Herpes simplex type II** (HSV-2)
- **Varicella-zoster virus** (VZV/HHV-3)
- **Epstein-Barr virus** (EBV/HHV-4)
- **Cytomegalovirus** (CMV/HHV-5)
- **Human herpesvirus type 6** (HBLV/HHV-6)
- **Human herpesvirus type 7** (HHV-7)
- **Kaposi's sarcoma herpesvirus** (KSHV/HHV-8).

They belong to the following three families:

Alpha-herpesviruses: HSV-1, HSV-2 and VZV – these have a relatively short reproductive cycle, variable host range, efficiently destroy infected cells and establish latent infections primarily in sensory ganglia.

Beta-herpesviruses: CMV, HHV-6 and HHV-7 – these have long reproductive cycles and a restricted host range. Infected cells often enlarge. Latency can be maintained in the white cells of the blood, kidneys, secretory glands and other tissues.

Gamma-herpesviruses: EBV and HHV-8 – these are specific for either T or B lymphocytes, and latency is often demonstrated in lymphoid tissue.

Symptoms

Signs of infection can present within 4 to 7 days after exposure, but sometimes it can be months or even years after getting infected before symptoms first appear.

- Blisters are the main symptom of herpes although many cases vary so patients may never get blisters, get them once, or they may come back now and again. Usually they are less painful and frequent over time
- Lethargy with flu-like aches and swollen glands
- Skin may itch, tingle or feel numb before blisters appear.

Treatment

Prescriptions for antiviral medications/topical creams will slow the progression of the virus rather than cure it.

- Use condoms if infected around genitals
- Wash your hands after touching blisters, especially before handling items such as contact lenses because herpes can cause eye infections
- Avoid factors which may aggravate herpes outbreaks such as a lack of sleep, sunbathing or stress
- Suppressive treatment may be used long-term by those who have more than six outbreaks in a year to manage symptoms, whereas other people may use episodic treatment when ever an outbreak occurs
- Pain-killing creams and bathing in salt water may help soothe blisters.

(THT, 2019)

Treatment plans for common herpes infections, such as **cold sores** and **chickenpox**, are covered in the following pages.

Chickenpox and shingles

Chickenpox in children

Chickenpox is a highly contagious infection caused by the **Varicella-zoster virus (VZV/HHV-3)**. A child with chickenpox is a common presentation in primary care but it is usually a self-limiting condition requiring minimal clinical intervention.

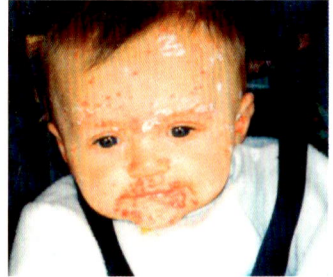

Symptoms

Chicken pox is characterised by low grade fever, malaise and maculopapular rash which then blisters and progresses to crusted lesions. The infection has an incubation period of 10–21 days. The child is infectious from 48 hours before the spots appear until all spots have crusted over (usually 5–7 days).

Treatment

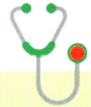

- Manage pyrexia
- Maintain fluids/hydration
- Application of **calamine lotion** may help ease the skin irritation
- Consider antihistamine medications
- Avoid exposure to pregnant women or elderly patients.

(NHS, 2017d; NICE, 2018j)

AVOID IBUPROFEN!

Ibuprofen suppresses the natural anti-inflammatory defence mechanism which can increase secondary bacterial risks.

IF a secondary infection is suspected then swab any pustule lesions and give flucloxacillin or amoxicillin.
If penicillin allergy then give clarithromycin.

Further assessment needed

- Pustules in eyes need immediate assessment
- Is the patient immunosuppressed?

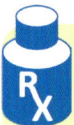

Check **BNF** dosage and local antimicrobial guidelines Aciclovir is the drug of choice for Varicella-zoster virus but is not routinely given to children with chickenpox. Immunocompromised or other complications will require GP to review.

Chickenpox in pregnancy

Most people have had chickenpox as a child therefore they have already developed immunity to it. Approximately 3 in 1,000 pregnant women in the UK will develop chickenpox and usually recover without a problem (NHS Inform, 2019c).

Pregnant women and neonates with chickenpox need to be clinically reviewed by a GP or suitably trained professional.

Complications with chickenpox during pregnancy can be fatal but this is very rare. Complications include (Harding, 2016b):

- **Pneumonia**
- **Encephalitis**
- **Hepatitis.**

Up to 28 weeks gestation

- **Mum** – no current evidence of increased risk of miscarriage
- **Baby** – possible risk of developing foetal varicella syndrome (FVS) which can affect the baby's skin, eyes, legs, arms, brain, bladder or bowel.

28 to 36 weeks gestation

The virus remains in the baby's body but is not symptomatic although the virus may become active in the first few years of life causing shingles.

36 weeks+gestation

Baby could be born with chickenpox or may contract chickenpox as a neonate if mum has new symptoms. Both will need medical assessment and treatment.

Shingles

After the initial infection of chickenpox the virus invades the nervous system and usually remains dormant for many years. However, it can reactivate as shingles (herpes zoster), The reactivation causes are unknown although stress, older age, HIV+ status and lower immunity are thought to be contributing factors (NHS Inform, 2019d).

Symptoms

- Pyrexia, lethargy, unwell
- Localised pain, burning, tingling, numbness or itchiness of the skin followed by a rash that develops into Itchy blister clusters
- The blister clusters follow a recognised nerve pathway without crossing the midline.

The rash can present in any area of the body including the face and eyes. The chest, back and abdomen are common sites.

Treatment

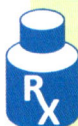

Check **BNF** dosage and local antimicrobial guidelines

<72 hours of the rash presentation then consider:

✔ **Aciclovir 800 mg 5 times a day for 7 days**

✔ Paracetamol and ibuprofen

✔ Maintain fluids/hydration

✔ Consider stronger analgesia for the pain such as codeine and monitor the skin for secondary infections.

(NICE, 2019i)

Further Reading

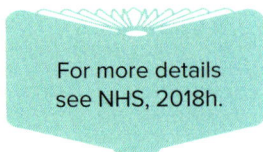

For more details see NHS, 2018h.

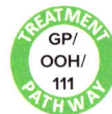

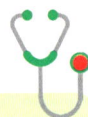

GP/
OOH/
111

Cold sores

Most cold sores are caused by **Herpes simplex type I (HSV-1)**.

Herpes simplex type II (HSV-2) is a different strain which causes genital herpes infections. HSV-1 is commonly passed on by skin contact such as kissing infected people and enters through the mucosa around the mouth. The virus is permanent and lies dormant in the nerve with no further symptoms although it may become active again due to being unwell, menstruation, stress or even from strong sunlight.

HSV-1 and -2 can cause lesions anywhere, so if a patient has oral sex a cold sore could be either strain.

Symptoms

Cold sores often start with a tingling, itching or burning sensation around the mouth. Small fluid-filled sores then appear, usually on the edges of the lower lip.

Further Reading

For more details see: NHS, 2017e.

Herpes simplex virus can also spread and cause local infections to broken skin, eczema or around the fingernails (herpetic whitlow).

Treatment

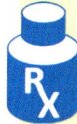

Check **BNF** dosage and local antimicrobial guidelines

<72 hours of presentation then consider:

✔ **Aciclovir topical cream**

Monitor the skin for secondary infections.

(NICE, 2016d)

OTC Variations of topical aciclovir are available from pharmacies

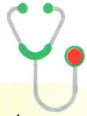

GP/ OOH/ 111

Monitor for any infection affecting the eye (**herpetic keratoconjunctivitis**) which requires immediate review.

Impetigo

This is usually a Staphylococcus aureus or Streptococcus pyogenes bacterial infection. The bacteria live within the nasal passages so the most common sites of infection are around the skin of the mouth and nose. This is a highly contagious condition mainly affecting children under 14 years of age and needs rapid treatment as it can easily contaminate other areas of the body via direct contact and shared towels (NICE, 2018k).

Symptoms

The spots develop into blisters (bullae) which then burst exposing a thick yellow discharge which covers the inflamed weeping area to form golden crusted lesions.

Bullous impetigo has much larger painful blisters which leave a very sore exposed wound over much larger areas.

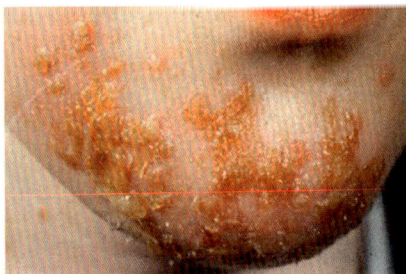

Treatment

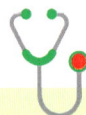

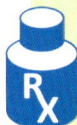

Check **BNF** dosage and local antimicrobial guidelines

✔ **Topical sodium fusidic acid TDS**
or
✔ **Flucloxacillin QDS**
✔ **Clarithromycin BD if allergy to flucloxacillin.**

(NICE, 2018k)

Crusts can be washed in warm water or mild soap and water with gentle removal of loose dried areas, dab the area dry with disposable paper towels. Encourage the child **NOT** to scratch at the blisters and lesions.

Advise that the child needs to stay away from school or nursery until the lesions have healed.

Further Reading

For more details see Knott, 2019.

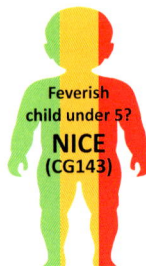

Feverish child under 5?
NICE
(CG143)

Insect bites and stings

- An **insect sting** is instantly painful and is followed by erythema and swelling (up to 1 cm) around the sting which resolves within a few hours.
- An **insect bite** may not give any symptoms initially. The saliva from the insect can cause skin irritation and become very itchy after time although some bites can still cause instant painful symptoms. Papules and wheals may also develop within 24 hours and last a few days with surrounding erythema.

Symptoms

- Itching rash which may spread away from the bite or sting
- Wheals/papules – blanching macular rash
- Patients are often concerned that this rash is infection but it is often an inflammatory histamine response.

- **Pyrexia or unwell systemically**
- **Cellulitis.**

Treatment

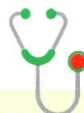

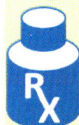

Check **BNF** dosage and local antimicrobial guidelines

✔ **Antihistamine** medications suitable to age and treatment plans

REMEMBER: Possible drowsy side effects of some medications

✔ **Consider flucloxacillin** or **clarithromycin** if secondary infection is suspected.

OTC

✔ **Manage pain with paracetamol, Ibuprofen and topical lidocaine gel.**

TREATMENT PATHWAY GP/ OOH/ 111

(NICE, 2016e)

See tick bites and Lyme disease on page 151.

Mosquito bites

The picture below shows a skin reaction to mosquito bites on the lower leg resulting in a severe localised reaction.

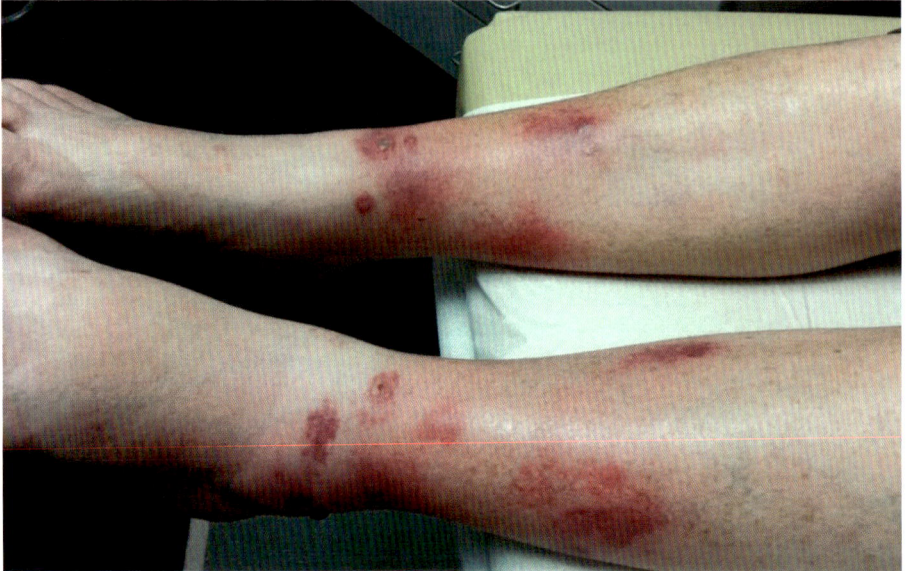

Symptoms

The itching rash had spread away from the bite entry with evidence of pustules and discharge forming on the right leg.

Peripheral circulation was satisfactory although the left foot was slightly swollen.

Treatment

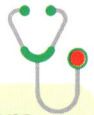

✔ **Antihistamine medications** were given and did ease the itching sensation

✔ **Prophylactic antibiotics** were also given in this case.

Keratosis pilaris (chicken skin)

Symptoms

The easiest way to remember or identify keratosis pilaris is to think of goose bumps. It is a common but harmless skin condition which presents as a fine but rough, permanent sandpaper-type rash very similar to goose bumps or, in fact, chicken skin, hence why it's sometimes known as chicken skin rash.

On occasions the skin patches can become inflamed and itch so there may be signs of redness or open areas of skin where the patient has scratched which are susceptible to infection.

- Keratosis pilaris is very common and affects one in three people in the UK of all ages
- It's very common in children and can improve or become worse during puberty but usually improves in adulthood.

(BAD, 2017)

The condition is hereditary and is not contagious to others.

Keratosis is the term for an excess of the protein keratin.

Keratin is an important protein within the epidermis but when an excess of keratin builds up around the hair follicles it causes a blockage resulting in plugs of hard, rough skin around the area. These blockages cause a widening of the skin pores and give the skin a thicker, spotty appearance (keratosis).

Keratosis pilaris is often associated with other dry, dermal conditions such as eczema and ichthyosis (genetic skin disorder) and will easily exacerbate the condition.

Treatment

Gentle exfoliation with a suitable pad or cloth may benefit.
There is no immediate treatment required unless there is an infection or itching becomes a problem. Treat dry areas of skin with emollients and advise antihistamines for itch relief (BAD, 2017c).

Lichen planus

Lichen refers to the small moss-like bumps on the skin and *planus* is Latin for 'flat top', This is a fairly common dermal condition which is a very itchy, non-infectious type of rash that usually affects adults. The cause is unknown although it is considered to be an immune system response (BAD, 2019).

Symptoms

The rash is made up of shiny, slightly raised purple spots with some lesions showing an irregular white streak (**Wickham's striae**) that lies on the flat, raised surface.

Common sites to be affected are:
- Fronts of the wrists and around the ankles
- Lower back
- Nails or the scalp
- Mouth – present in about 30–70% of those who have it on their skin.

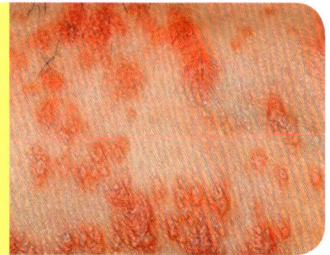

Treatment

There is no cure for lichen planus and it usually improves on its own although this can take up to 18 months to resolve. Body areas involving hair or nails can last much longer and darker Asian or Afro-Caribbean skin can be left with pigmented stains to the skin Topical steroids can be used to treat the intense itching (PCDS, 2018c).

The genital area can also be affected and cause some purple or white ring-shaped patches although they generally do not cause such an intense itching sensation.

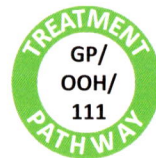

TREATMENT PATHWAY
GP/ OOH/ 111

Lyme disease

Lyme borreliosis (Lyme disease) is caused by the bacteria Borrelia burgdorferi and is spread by tick bites. Only a small number of ticks are infected with the bacteria and they can only cause Lyme disease in humans if the tick has already bitten an infected animal. From the bite entry site on the skin, the bacteria can travel to various parts of the body and cause inflammation of the joints and tissues. The tick must be attached for 36 to 48 hours before the bacteria can really spread (CDC, 2019). The most common sign of infection is an expanding area of redness on the skin, known as erythema migrans.

Symptoms

Erythema migrans begins at the site of the bite after approximately 7 days. The rash itself is usually asymptomatic and not all infections will cause this rash.

Contributing symptoms are lethargy and pyrexia. Later symptoms include shooting pains or tingling in the arms and legs.

Despite appropriate treatment, about 10 to 20% of people develop joint pains, memory problems and feel tired for at least 6 months.

Months to years later, repeated episodes of joint pain and swelling may occur.

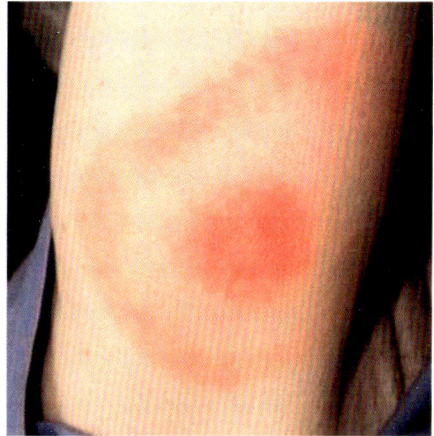

Further Reading

For more details on tick bites and the prevention of Lyme disease see Public Health England, 2018b and CDC, 2019.

Treatment

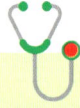

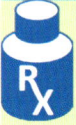

Check **BNF** for dosage and local antimicrobial guidelines. For details visit https://cks.nice.org.uk/lyme-disease#!scenario

For adults and children 12 years of age or older:

✔ **First-line — doxycycline**
100 mg 2 x daily (contraindicated in pregnancy and if breastfeeding) or **amoxicillin** 500 mg 3 x daily (off-label use)

✔ **Second-line — cefuroxime axetil 500 mg twice daily.**

For children younger than 12 years of age:

✔ **First line — amoxicillin:**
500 mg 3 x daily for children aged 5–12 years old
250 mg 3 x daily for children aged 1 year–4 years 11 months
125 mg 3 x daily for children aged 1–11 months old

✔ **Second line — cefuroxime axetil:**
15 mg/kg (maximum of 500 mg per dose) twice daily for children aged 3 months – 12 years.

How to remove a tick

1. Grasp tick with fine head tweezers close to skin.
2. Pull upward with steady, even pressure. **Don't twist or jerk** as this may cause mouth-parts to remain in the skin. Should this happen, use the tweezers to remove the mouth parts. If removing the mouth parts is not easily achieved using the tweezers then leave it alone and let the skin heal.
3. Clean the bite area and wash your hands once the tick is removed.
4. Dispose of a live tick by submersing it in alcohol, placing it in a sealed bag/container, wrapping it tightly in tape, or flushing it down the toilet.
   Never crush a tick with your fingers.

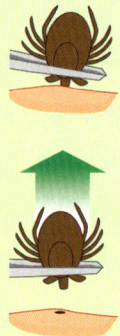

(CDC, 2019)

Molluscum contagiosum

Molluscum contagiosum can occur at any age but most commonly affects children (NHS, 2017e).

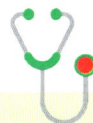

Symptoms

A common localised poxvirus infection causing small round lesions mainly on the trunk and back which can take about 18 months to clear. In isolation, these lesions will not cause illness and are of little clinical concern although if picked or knocked they may cause a local secondary infection. The spots are not usually painful but can be itchy. Parents may be concerned about the risk of scarring but the risk is normally very low.

Treatment

Self-limiting condition resolving within 18 months. The child may complain of itching at times which can be treated with antihistamine medications.

Children and parents may become very aware/self-conscious of the condition leading to anxiety.

If a secondary infection occurs due to one spot being picked or knocked then consider topical treatments or oral antibiotics

(NHS, 2017e)

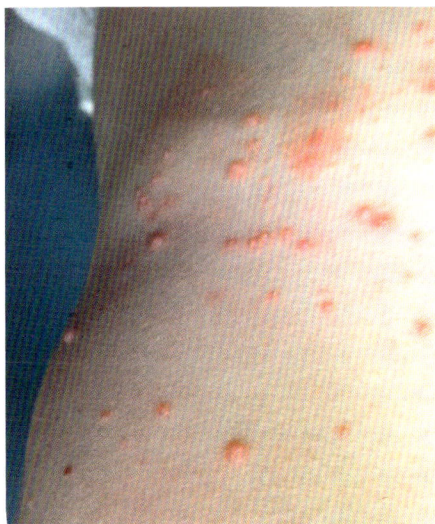

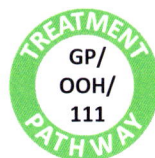

TREATMENT PATHWAY
GP/
OOH/
111

Paronychia (whitlow)

An **acute paronychia** or whitlow is an infection of the skin folds (paronychium) around the nail bed and can be caused by either a bacterial (Staphylococcus aureus), fungal or herpes-type virus.

A **chronic paronychia** is usually a gradual process which can start in one of the proximal nail folds then spread laterally to infect other fingers. Each affected nail fold is swollen and tends to lift off the nail plat. It can also be thickened, distorted and develop transverse ridges.

Symptoms

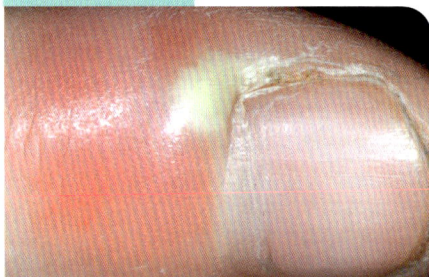

Symptoms are pain, redness and swelling of the finger pulp and nail folds.

Pus may be evident and can increase to a larger cyst with more severe infections.

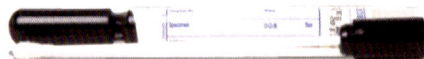

Treatment

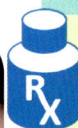

Check **BNF** dosage and local antimicrobial guidelines

For acute minor localised infections consider:
✔ **Topical fusidic acid**
If pus or swollen pulp consider oral antibiotics:
✔ **Flucloxacillin** or **clarithromycin** (if known allergy to penicillin)
✔ **Consider aciclovir** if suspected herpes simplex infection.

Surgical incision, drainage and irrigation may be required for larger infections, then packed with gauze.

Advise the patient to soak affected finger in warm salt water several times a day.

Consider swab and send for fungal culture.

(NICE, 2017a)

Rosacea

Rosacea usually affects about 1 in 10 middle-aged people in the UK with presentation of a red rash affecting the face, nose, cheeks and forehead although other areas, such as the neck, chest and ears can be affected. Most cases are mild clinically although distress and self-awareness can be additional issues for the patient (PCDS, 2018b).

Symptoms

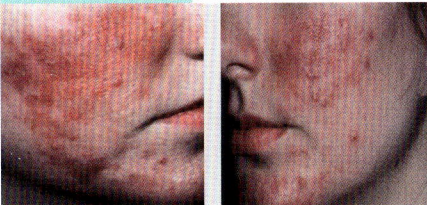

- **Frequent flushing** is an early symptom seen for months or years before anything else develops
- **Erythema** (redness) patches
- **Papules** or pustules which look similar to acne
- **Telangectasia** – blood vessels cause thread like red lines or patterns on skin
- **Eye symptoms** (ocular rosacea) occur in about half of cases but are often mild. They can include:
  - Sensation of something in the eye
  - Burning, stinging, itchy eyes
  - Dry eyes
  - Sensitivity to light.

Treatment

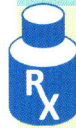 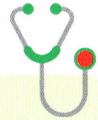

Check **BNF** dosage and local antimicrobial guidelines

Topical treatments

Mild symptoms: Soolantra® (ivermectin 10 mg/g) cream OD for up to 4 months, Rozex® (metronidazole 0.75%) gel or cream BD, or Finacea® (azelaic acid 15%) cream BD.

Systemic treatments

Use if topical applications fail or more severe symptoms occur. Both oral medications are taken on an empty stomach.

✔ Doxycycline 40 mg OD

✔ Erythromycin 500 mg BD is an alternative

Initial treatment should be for at least 3 months, although if the patient is responding well the dose may be reduced after 1 month.

(PCDS, 2018b)

Scabies

Scabies is caused by a tiny parasite mite called Sarcoptes scabiei. The female mites tunnel into the skin and lay around 50 eggs during their life cycle. These hatch into larvae after 3–4 days and take around 10–15 days to mature to adults. The intense itching symptoms of scabies are due to an immune response to the parasites, saliva and faeces (Starr, 2017).

Contrary to popular belief scabies mites cannot jump or fly but they can be passed via prolonged skin contact such as holding hands.

Symptoms

Intense itching!

Note the burrow pattern

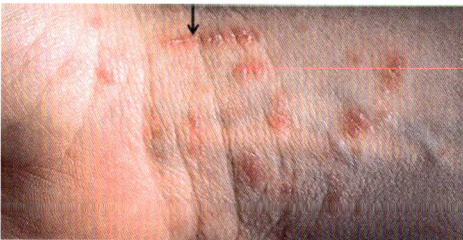

Common sites of infection

Mites are often found between fingers and on wrists.

Pink areas show common sites of rashes.

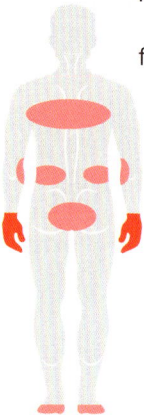

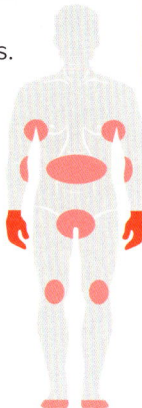

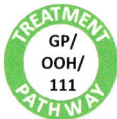

TREATMENT
GP/
OOH/
111
PATHWAY

Treatment

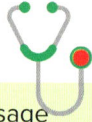

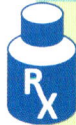

Check **BNF** dosage and local antimicrobial guidelines

Treat the whole body

Advise special cleaning attention under nails

✔ **Permethrin 5% cream**
2 applications 7 days apart.

If allergy to permethrin then:

✔ **Malathion 0.5% aqueous liquid**
2 applications 7 days apart.

(Starr, 2017)

Scarlet fever

This is a bacterial infection caused by group A Streptococcus. Historically this was considered a dangerous infection but since the use of antibiotics it has now become much less of a concern.

Symptoms

- Sore throat
- Tender lymph nodes
- Pyrexia and lethargy
- Tonsils may be swollen, red or exudate evident.

A blanching **'fine sandpaper rash'** develops around the face and trunk.

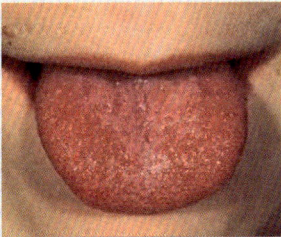

The tongue initially has a white coating which peels to reveal a bright red (strawberry) appearance after 5 days.

Treatment

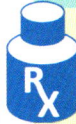

Check **BNF** for correct dosage and local antimicrobial guidelines

✔ **Phenoxymethylpenicillin (Penicillin V) QDS for 10 days** or **amoxicillin** for 10 days if unable to tolerate Penicillin V.

If allergy to penicillin:

✔ **Clarithromycin 5–7 days.**

OTC

Manage pyrexia with paracetamol and ibuprofen

Maintain fluids/hydration.

(NICE, 2018m)

Notifiable disease in England and Wales
Inform local health protection teams of suspected cases

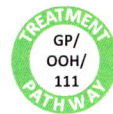

TREATMENT PATHWAY

GP/ OOH/ 111

157

Seborrhoeic keratosis

There is no known cause of seborrhoeic keratosis but it is a common skin complaint in primary care, with the patient having concerns of cancer. It presents at any age although it tends to be more prominent at age 50+. Common sites affected are face, chest, shoulders or the back/flank presenting as a single growth or cluster (Mayo Clinic, 2019c).

Seborrhoeic keratosis doesn't usually cause any pain but depending on where the lesions are they can be damaged by dressing, showering or the toils of everyday life so they are susceptible to infection if damage occurs.

Symptoms

- A waxy wart-type of growth
- Varies in colour, from light tan to brown or black
- Is round or oval shaped
- Ranges in size
- May itch if damaged.

Acute multiple growths

Sores that bleed or fail to heal

These could be signs of skin cancer!

Treatment

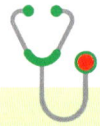

If the lesions are not cancerous and cause no irritation then no immediate treatment or removal is required. Several methods of removal are:

- **Cryotherapy** – freezing with liquid nitrogen
- **Electrocautery** – burning using an electric current
- **Curettage** – surgical shaving of the skin.

(Mayo Clinic, 2019c)

Depending on your clinical experience and confidence then a second opinion from a GP or specialist to confirm the diagnosis or consider further investigations and treatment plans is **always a wise decision!**

Slapped cheek

Alternative titles for this infection are **erythema infectiosum** or **fifth disease**. This is caused by parvovirus B19 and is most common in age groups from 2–12 years, although adults can contract it. Pregnant women with parvovirus B19 infection require GP to review for further tests and treatment plan to exclude rubella. This infection has an incubation period of around 13–18 days and is infective until the rash appears (NICE, 2017a).

Symptoms

Symptoms include bright red rash on cheeks (hence 'slapped cheek') which may spread to arms and trunk.

Joint pains are common in adults and additional pyrexia, runny nose and diarrhoea may be present.

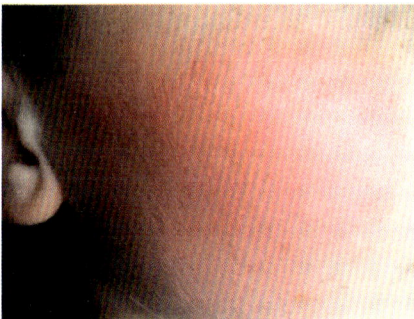

Treatment

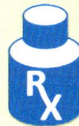 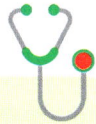

Check **BNF** for correct dosage and local guidelines

No immediate treatment required although paracetamol and ibuprofen can be given for pyrexia and joint pains.

No exclusion from school is required unless diarrhoea is present.

(NICE, 2017a)

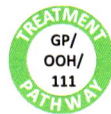

GP/
OOH/
111

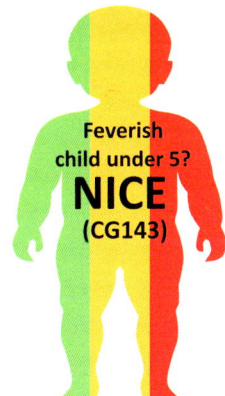

Feverish
child under 5?
NICE
(CG143)

🚩 Pregnant patients require GP referral

159

Urticaria (nettle rash)

This is another quite dramatic-looking rash which is an immune system response to either infection or allergy. **Idiopathic urticaria** is when there is an unknown source of the reaction response. Urticaria can vary in duration. **Acute urticaria** is any reaction lasting less than 6 weeks where as **chronic urticaria** is any reaction lasting more than 6 weeks. Consider a follow-up appointment with a GP if symptoms are not improving.

Symptoms

Usually this has a very rapid onset causing a widespread, very itchy red rash with wheals (hives) due to the dilation of the capillaries and the release of histamine from the mast cells or basophils.

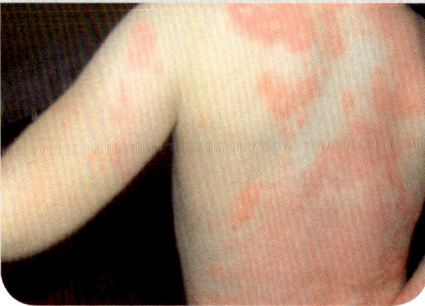

AVOID NSAIDS
as this will exacerbate the rash.

Treatment

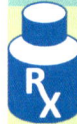

Check **BNF** for correct dosage and local guidelines

Oral antihistamines such as cetirizine or loratadine can help ease the irritation of itching.

✔ **Chlorphenamine** (may cause a drowsy side effect)
✔ For idiopathic urticaria give **fexofenadine for children over 12 years old.**

Blood tests for chronic urticaria
FBC; CRP/ESR; Thyroid antibodies; anti-TTG/ANA.

Patch testing will not benefit the condition or diagnosis.

(NICE, 2018n)

GP/ OOH/ 111

Vasculitis

The causes of vasculitis are generally unknown but the condition will stimulate the immune system to attack the blood vessels causing an inflammation. This in turn interrupts blood flow affecting delivery of oxygen, nutrients etc. to the tissues and removal of waste products.

The symptoms of vasculitis vary greatly depending on which type of blood vessels have been affected and which organs they supply.

Vasculitis examples

Eosinophilic granulomatosis with polyangiitis (Churg-Strauss syndrome)
A type of vasculitis that mainly affects adults aged 30 to 45.

Granulomatosis with polyangiitis (Wegener's granulomatosis)
A type of vasculitis that mainly affects blood vessels in the nose, sinuses, ears, lungs and kidneys. Usually affects middle-aged or elderly people.

Giant cell arteritis (temporal arteritis)
Giant cell arteritis is a type of vasculitis that often affects the arteries in the head and neck mostly occurring in adults over the age of 50.

Less common examples of vasculitis are:

■ **Henoch-Schönlein purpura**
  – see page 139

■ **Kawasaki disease**

■ **Microscopic polyangiitis**

■ **Polyarteritis nodosa.**

Further Reading

For more detailed information on each of these vasculitis variations see NHS, 2019c.

Symptoms

- Early common vasculitis symptoms include malaise and aching joints and may have been preceded by a primary infection such as a common cold and pyrexia

- Dermal or soft tissue vasculitis can cause petechial/purpuric rashes and pain

- Pulmonary vasculitis can cause shortness of breath and lead to haemoptysis

- Renal vasculitis can lead to haematuria and renal failure.

Treatment

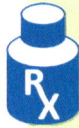

Discuss diagnosis and plan with the duty doctor

- Obtain a **urine sample** if possible and test for infection, blood etc.

- **Obtain a stool sample** if possible, monitoring for blood

- **Monitor blood pressure**

- Has a recent medication caused these symptoms? If yes then stop.

(PCDS, 2019d)

Initially admission to hospital is likely followed by regular monitoring of blood pressure in GP practice. Urinalysis may also form part of a chronic plan.

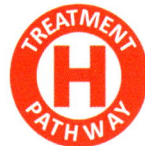

Viral rashes

A viral rash has no clear or specific characteristics so it is more likely associated with a history of generalised symptoms such as pyrexia or cough. If the symptoms are mild then the rash is usually not too concerning and should settle within a few days. There is no specific treatment for the rash itself although antihistamine medication is a consideration for any itching along with paracetamol for the pyrexia (Newson, 2016). Eczema or urticaria can also cause very similar presentations to viral rashes.

Symptoms

- Rashes vary in shape and colour
- Affect most of the body surface
- Acute presentation lasting a few days
- Resolves quickly
- Associated symptoms such as pyrexia
- May be itchy.

Treatment

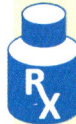

Check **BNF** for correct dosage and local guidelines

✔ **Paracetamol**

✔ **Antihistamines**

✔ **Calamine lotion MAY benefit.**

OTC

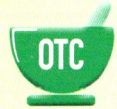

The source of the infection may not always be evident. Consider any secondary infection risks and treat accordingly.

(Newson, 2016)

An acute dramatic-looking rash associated with mild clinical symptoms will usually resolve quickly.

Always consider sepsis/ meningitis risk

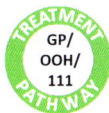

TREATMENT PATHWAY
GP/ OOH/ 111

Vitiligo

Symptoms

Vitiligo is a condition where pale white patches develop on the skin due to a lack of pigment in the affected areas.

There are very few melanocytes left in the skin area as they have been damaged or destroyed resulting in no production of melanin to colour and protect the skin. It is not clear why the melanocytes are lost but they may be destroyed by an autoimmune condition or malfunction.

The appearance of vitiligo can be distressing particularly for patients with darker skin where white patches are more noticeable. About 1 in 100 people develop vitiligo, both men and women are equally affected and it is not more common in any racial or ethnic groups.

It can develop at any age although it tends to begin before the age of 20 years in about half of cases. There are some genetic factors involved and vitiligo may run in the family, so statistically nearly 1 in 3 affected people have some other family member who is also affected (Harding, 2016c).

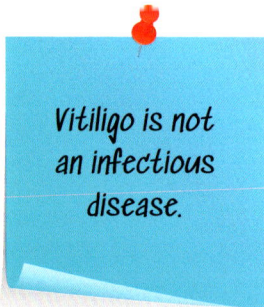

Vitiligo is not an infectious disease.

Treatment

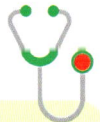

There is no known cure for vitiligo and the affected skin patches are usually permanent, however, there are cases where the skin pigmentation has returned to some degree. There are a number of alternative treatment options which would need to be discussed with the patient's GP but there is no guarantee of success. SPF protection should, however, be used by those affected. No melanin, no protection (Harding, 2016c).

Warts and verrucas

Warts and verrucas are caused through direct contact with HPV and they are contagious, often spreading by direct contact or through contact with floor surfaces such as swimming pools. Warts and verrucas will vary depending on which HPV virus is responsible and where it has grown.

A HPV infection is caused by human papillomavirus and there are over 130 identified types. HPV causes an excess amount of keratin which then stimulates rapid growth of cells within the epidermis.

Common wart (Verruca vulgaris) is a raised growth with rough surfaces and are most common on the hands

Flat wart (Verruca plana) is a small, smooth, flat wart which is flesh-coloured and can occur in clusters. They are most common on the face, neck, hands, wrists and knees

Filiform or **digitate wart** is a thread-like wart, most common on the face, especially near the eyelids and lips

Genital wart occurs on the genitalia

Periungual wart is a cauliflower-like cluster of warts that occurs around the nails

Plantar wart (Verruca plantaris) is a hard, sometimes painful lump, often with multiple black specks in the centre, usually only found on pressure points on the soles of the feet

Mosaic wart is a group of tightly clustered plantar-type warts, commonly on the hands or soles of the feet.

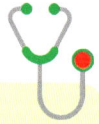

Symptoms

Warts

- Oval-shaped, usually firm and raised with a rough, irregular surface similar to a cauliflower surface
- They vary in size, from less than 1 mm to more than 1 cm across
- Appear singularly or in groups.

Verrucas

- Develop on the soles of the feet and can be painful if they're on a weight-bearing area
- Appearance is usually white with a black dot in the centre
- They are flat rather than raised.

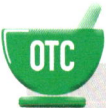

OTC

Many varied preparations within different price ranges

Treatment

Most types of warts will resolve without treatment – this may take months to years.

- **Freezing (cryotherapy):** liquid nitrogen freezes the infection and kills the cells. Often takes several applications and is not always successful
- **Salicylic acid:** 'burns' off the top layer of the wart then requires the dead tissue to be rubbed away with an emery board or similar
- **Duct tape:** strong adhesive tape removes the top layers of skin slowly. This is not recommended for warts but can be used for verrucas on feet.

Difficult or problematic growths can sometimes be considered for laser or minor surgery if all other treatments have failed.

(NICE, 2014; BAD, 2018)

A–Z of common skin conditions

Acne

The most common skin condition, affects over 85% of people at some time in life

Actinic keratosis

A crusty or scaly bump that forms on sun-exposed skin. Actinic keratosis can sometimes progress to cancer

Angiogenesis

Development of new blood vessels

Autolytic debridement

Selective to necrotic tissue

Basal cell carcinoma

The most common type of skin cancer

Cellulitis

Inflammation of dermis and subcutaneous tissues, usually due to an infection

Dandruff

A scaly condition of scalp caused by seborrhoeic dermatitis, psoriasis or eczema

Dermatitis

A general term for inflammation of the skin. Atopic dermatitis (a type of eczema) is the most common form

Eczema

Skin inflammation (dermatitis) causing an itchy rash. Most often, it's due to an overactive immune system

Herpes

The herpes viruses HSV-1 and HSV-2 can cause periodic blisters or skin irritation around the lips or the genitals

Hives

Raised, red, itchy patches on the skin that arise suddenly. Hives usually result from an allergic reaction

Melanoma

The most dangerous type of skin cancer, melanoma results from sun damage and other causes

Psoriasis

An autoimmune condition that can cause a variety of skin rashes. Silver, scaly plaques on the skin are the most common form

Rash

Nearly any change in the skin's appearance can be called a rash. Most rashes are from simple skin irritation; others result from medical conditions

Ringworm
A fungal skin infection (also called tinea)

Rosacea
A chronic skin condition causing a red rash on the face

Scabies
Tiny mites that burrow into the skin cause scabies. An intensely itchy rash in the webs of fingers, wrists, elbows, and buttocks is typical of scabies

Seborrhoeic keratosis
A benign, often itchy growth that appears like a 'stuck-on' wart

Shingles
Herpes zoster: caused by the chickenpox virus, shingles is a painful rash on one side of the body

Skin abscess
Boil or furuncle: localised skin infection – a collection of pus under skin

Squamous cell carcinoma
A common form of skin cancer, squamous cell carcinoma may begin as an ulcer that won't heal, or an abnormal growth. It usually develops in sun-exposed areas

Tinea versicolor
Benign fungal skin infection – pale areas of low pigmentation on skin

Viral exantham
Many viral infections can cause a red rash affecting large areas of the skin. This is especially common in children

Warts
A virus infects the skin and causes the skin to grow excessively

For a list of **terminology to use when describing skin conditions** see pages 60–64.

References

AAD (2019). Nummular Dermatitis. *American Academy of Dermatology Associatation*. Available at: https://www.aad.org/nummular-eczema [Accessed: 11 December 2019].

ABPI (2019). Code of Practice for the Pharmaceutical Industry. *The Association of the British Pharmaceutical Industry*. Available at:https://www.abpi.org.uk/publications/code-of-practice-for-the-pharmaceutical-industry-2019/ [Accessed: 27 August 2019].

Aderibigbe BA and Buyana B (2018). Alginate in wound dressings. *Pharmaceutics*. Available at: https://www.ncbi.nlm.nih.gov/pmc/articles/PMC6027439/ [Accessed: 10 December 2019].

Advanced Tissue (2014). Your guide to hydrocolloid dressings. Available at: https://advancedtissue.com/2014/12/guide-hydrocolloid-dressings/ [Accessed: 10 December 2019].

Alendar F et al. (2009). Early detection of melanoma skin cancer. *Bosnian Journal of Basic Medical Sciences*, 9(1): 77–80. [Accessed: 28 March 2019].

American Cancer Society (2016). What causes melanoma skin cancer? Available at: https://www.cancer.org/cancer/melanoma-skin-cancer/causes-risks-prevention/what-causes.html [Accessed: 28 March 2019].

BAD (2014). Lentigo maligna. *British Association of Dermatologists*. Available at: http://www.bad.org.uk/shared/get-file.ashx?id=1907&itemtype=document [Accessed: 28 March 2019].

BAD (2015). The British Association of Dermatologists' information on topical corticosteroids – established and alternative proprietary names, potency, and discontinuation. *British Association of Dermatologists*. Available at: http://www.bad.org.uk/shared/get-file.ashx?id=3427&itemtype=document [Accessed: 27 August 2019].

BAD (2016). Actinic Keratoses – also known as solar keratoses. *British Association of Dermatologists*. Available at: http://www.bad.org.uk/for-the-public/patient-information-leaflets/actinic-keratoses/?showmore=1&returnlink=http%3a%2f%2fwww.bad.org.uk%2fforthe public%2fpatient-information-leaflets#.XZozMy2ZOqQ [Accessed: 27 August 2019].

BAD (2017a). Contact dermatitis. *British Association of Dermatologists*. Available at: http://www.bad.org.uk/for-the-public/patient-information-leaflets/contactdermatitis/?showmore=1&returnlink=http%3a%2f%2fwww.bad.org.uk%2fforthe-public%2fpatient-information-leaflets#.Xah7ZehKiUk [Accessed: 24 July 2019].

BAD (2017b). Head Lice. *The British Association of Dermatologists*. Available at: https://www.provide.org.uk/resources/uploads/files/Head%20lice.pdf [Accessed: 11 December 2019].

BAD (2017c). Keratosis Pilaris. *The British Association of Dermatologists*. Available at: https://www.provide.org.uk/resources/uploads/files/Head%20lice.pdf [Accessed: 12 December 2019].

BAD (2017d). Tinea Capitis. *British Association of Dermatologists*. Available at: http://www.bad.org.uk/ResourceListing. aspx?sitesectionid=159&itemid=1201 [Accessed: 12 December 2019].

BAD (2018). Plantar warts (verrucas). *British Association of Dermatologists*. Available at: http://www.bad.org.uk/shared/get-file.ashx?id=176&itemtype=document [Accessed: 14 January 2020].

BAD (2019a). Discoid eczema. *British Association of Dermatologists*. Available at: http://www.bad.org.uk/shared/get-file.ashx?id=80&itemtype=document [Accessed: 12 December 2019].

BAD (2019b). Lichen Planus. *The British Association of Dermatologists*. Available at: http://www.bad.org.uk/for-the-public/patient-information-leaflets/lichen-planus/?showmore=1&returnlink=http%3a%2f%2fwww.bad.org.uk%2ffor-the-public%2fpatient-information-leaflets#.XfI2I-j7SUI [Accessed: 12 December 2019].

Baidya S (2015). 50 interesting human skin facts. Available at: https://factslegend.org/50-interesting-human-skin-facts/ [Accessed: 24 July 2019].

Baxter H (2013). Management of surgical wounds. *Nursing Times*. Available at: https:/ www.nursingtimes.net/clinical-archive/tissue-viability/management-of-surgical-wounds-01-04-2003/ [Accessed: 10 December 2019].

Bewley T et al. (2015). Acne – Primary care. *Primary Care Dermatology Society*. Available at: http:// www.pcds.org.uk/ee/images/uploads/general/Acne_Treatment_2015-web.pdf [Accessed: 28 March 2019].

BNF (British National Formulary (2017). *BNF 73*. London: Pharmaceutical Press.

British Skin Foundation (2016). Melanoma. Available at: https://www.britishskinfoundation.org.uk/ melanomaskincancer [Accessed: 28 March 2019].

British Skin Foundation (2019a). Contact Dermatitis. Available at: https://www.britishskinfoundation. org.uk/contact-dermatitis?gclid=CjwKCAiA58fvBRAzEiwAQW-hzd5kSxH30E1SyYRHeU-CxqIQMj9YOJw6QMunfFzoBllsz7kIQKY4vBoCs4wQAvD_BwE [Accessed: 12 December 2019].

British Skin Foundation (2019b). Acne. Available at: https://www.britishskinfoundation.org.uk/acne [Accessed: 27 August 2019].

Buchweitz O (2016). Cosmetic outcome of skin adhesives versus transcutaneous sutures in laparoscopic port-site wounds: a prospective randomized controlled trial. *Surgical Endoscopy*, 30(6): 2326–2331.

Cancer Research UK (2015). Clark and Breslow staging. Available at: https://www.cancerresearchuk. org/about-cancer/melanoma/stages-types/clark-breslow-staging [Accessed: 28 March 2019].

Cancer Research UK (2017). Skin cancer: types. Available at: https://www.cancerresearchuk.org/ about-cancer/skin-cancer/types [Accessed: 28 March 2019].

Cancer Research UK (2019). Melanoma skin cancer statistics. Available at: https://www. cancerresearchuk.org/health-professional/cancer-statistics/statistics-by-cancer-type/ melanoma-skin-cancer#heading-Zero [Accessed: 28 March 2019].

CDC (2010d). Facts about 'hot tub rash' and 'swimmer's ear' (pseudomonas). *Centers for Disease Control and Prevention*. Available at: https://www.cdc.gov/healthywater/pdf/swimming/ resources/pseudomonas-factsheet.pdf. [Accessed: 28 November 2019].

CDC (2016b). What are the Risk Factors for Skin Cancer? *Centers for Disease Control and Prevention*. Available at: https://www.cdc.gov/cancer/skin/basic_info/risk_factors.htm [Accessed: 28 March 2019].

CDC (2019). Lyme disease. Centers for *Disease Control and Prevention*. Available at: https://www. cdc.gov/lyme/transmission/index.html. [Accessed: 12 December 2019].

CIRS (2016). EU Public Consultation on Methylisothiazolinone (MI) Ban for Leave-on Cosmetic Products Launched. Available at: http://www.cirs-reach.com/news-and-articles/eu-public-consultation-on-methylisothiazolinone-mi-ban-for-leave-on-cosmetic-products-launched. html [Accessed: 28 March 2019].

Colantonio S, Bracken MB and Beeker J (2014). The association of indoor tanning and melanoma in adults: systematic review and meta-analysis. *Journal of the American Academy of Dermatology*, 70(5): 847–857.

Coloplast (2013). Wound Healing – Mode of Action. Available at: https://www.youtube.com/ watch?v=RiKu9sgFizYandt=4s [Accessed: 24 July 2019].

Cormack D (2001). *Essential Histology*. Lippincott Williams & Wilkins.

D'Ath P and Thompson P (2012). Superficial spreading melanoma. *BMJ*, 334: 2319.

Dawson AL and Dellavalle RP (2013). Acne Vulgaris. *BMJ*, 345: f2634.

Dermapak (2018). Instructions for Dermapak Type 4. Available at: https://www.dermapak.net/ [Accessed: 27 August 2019].

Divya S, Padma VV, Santhini E (2015). Wound dressings - a review. *Biomedicine*, 5(4): 22.

Eske (2019). 10 natural remedies for dandruff. *Medical News Today*. Available at: https://www.medicalnewstoday.com/articles/324756.php [Accessed: 28 November 2019].

European Commission (2016). Commission Regulation (EU) 2016/1198 of 22 July 2016 amending Annex V to Regulation (EC) No 1223/2009 of the European Parliament and of the Council on cosmetic products (Text with EEA relevance). C/2016/4622 OJ L 198, 23.7.2016, p. 10 –12. Available at: https://eur-lex.europa.eu/legal-content/EN/XT/?uri=CELEX%3A32016R1198 [Accessed: 25 August 2019].

Farage MA et al. (2013). Characteristics of the Aging Skin. *Advanced Wound Care*, 2(1): 5–10.

Forefront Dermatology (2017). *Skin Fun Facts*. Available at: https://forefrontdermatology.com/skin-fun-facts/ [Accessed: 24 July 2019].

Foster KG, Hey EN and Katz G (1969). The response of the sweat glands of the newborn baby to thermal stimuli and to intradermal acetylcholine. *Journal of Physiology*, 203(1): 13–29.

Gallagher RP and Lee TK (2006). Adverse effects of ultraviolet radiation: a brief review. *Progress in Biophysics and Molecular Biology*, (92): 119–131.

Gandini S et al. (2005). Meta-analysis of risk factors for cutaneous melanoma: II. Sun exposure. *European Journal of Cancer*, 41: 45–60.

Grice EA, Kong HH, Conlan S (2009). Topographical and temporal diversity of the human skin microbiome. *Science*, 324 (5931): 1190–1192.

Guinness H (2018). *Anatomy and Physiology* (5th ed.). London: Hodder Education.

Harding M (2014). Contact and occupational dermatitis. *Patient*. Available at: https://patient.info/doctor/Contact-and-Occupational-Dermatitis [Accessed: 25 July 2019].

Harding M (2016a). Pityriasis Rosea. *Patient*. Available at: https://patient.info/childrens-health/viral-skin-infections-leaflet/pityriasisrosea [Accessed: 28 March 2019].

Harding M (2016b). Chickenpox contact in pregnancy. *Patient*. Available at: https://patient.info/pregnancy/pregnancy-complications/chickenpox-contact-in-pregnancy [Accessed: 28 March 2019].

Harding M (2016c). Vitiligo. *Patient*. Available at: https://patient.info/doctor/vitiligo-pro [Accessed: 28 March 2019].

Harvard Medical School (2019). Blisters (Overview). Available at: https://www.health.harvard.edu/a_to_z/blisters-overview-a-to-z. [Accessed: 20 November 2019].

Healsmith MF et al. (1994). An evaluation of the revised seven-point checklist for the early diagnosis of cutaneous malignant melanoma. *British Journal of Dermatology*, 130(1): 48–50.

Higuera V (2019). What is cellulitis. *Everyday Health*. Available at: https://www.everydayhealth.com/cellulitis/guide/ [Accessed: 11 December 2019].

Holmes TR (2019) Removing stitches (sutures). *eMedicineHealth*. Available at: https://www.emedicinehealth.com/removing_stitches/article_em.htm#facts_you_should_know_about_removing_stitches_sutures [Accessed: 15 January 2019].

HPA (2008). Guidance on the diagnosis and management of PVL-associated staphylococcus aureus infections (PVL-SA) in England. *Health Protection Agency*, Available at: https://assets.publishing.service.gov.uk/government/uploads/system/uploads/attachment_data/file/322857/Guidance_on_the_diagnosis_and_management_of_PVL_associated_SA_infections_in_England_2_Ed.pdf [Accessed: 24 July 2019].

Irmak MK, Oztas E and Vural H (2004). Dependence of fetal hairs and sebaceous glands on fetal adrenal cortex and possible control from adrenal medulla. *Medical Hypotheses*, 62(4): 486–492.

James W et al. (2019). *Andrews' Diseases of the Skin: Clinical Dermatology* (13th ed.) Philadelphia: Saunders.

Kalkhoran S et al. (2010). Historical, clinical and dermoscopic characteristics of thin nodular melanoma. *Archives of Dermatology*, 146(3): 311–318.

Knott L (2017). Folliculitis. *Patient*. Available at: https://patient.info/doctor/folliculitis-pro [Accessed: 12 December 2019].

Knott L (2019). Impetigo. *Patient*. Available at: https://patient.info/childrens-health/impetigo-leaflet [Accessed: 28 March 2019].

Leiter U et al. (2008). Epidemiology of melanoma and nonmelanoma ski cancer – the role of sunlight. *Advances in Experimental Medicine and Biology*, 624: 89–103.

Levinson, W et al. (2010). *Review of Medical Microbiology and Immunology* (15th ed.) New York: McGraw-Hill Education.

Likness LP (2011). Common dermatologic infections in athletes and return-to-play guidelines. *The Journal of the American Osteopathic Association*, 111(6): 373–379.

Loewenstein M (2016). All you need to know about caring for your Afro. *Woman&Home*. Availble at: https://www.womanandhomemagazine.co.za/beauty/hair/afro [Accessed: 10 December 2019].

Marieb E and Hoehn K (2015). *Human Anatomy & Physiology, Global Edition* (10th ed.) London: Pearson.

Marsden JR, et al. (2010). Revised UK guidelines for the management of cutaneous melanoma 2010. *Journal of Plastic, Reconstructive and Aesthetic Surgery*, 63(9): 1401–1419.

Mayo Clinic (2019a). Staph Infections. Available at: https://www.mayoclinic.org/diseasesconditions/staph-infections/symptomscauses/syc-20356221 [Accessed: 24 July 2019].

Mayo Clinicnot (2019b). Nail fungus. Available at: https://www.mayoclinic.org/diseases-conditions/nail-fungus/symptoms-causes/syc-20353294 [Accessed: 12 December 2019].

Mayo Clinic (2019c). Seborrheic keratosis. Available at: https://www.mayoclinic.org/diseases-conditions/seborrheic-keratosis/symptoms-causes/syc-20353878 [Accessed: 12 December 2019].

McGrath JA and Uitto J (2016). Structure and Function the Human Skin. In Griffiths C et al. (eds.). *Rook's Textbook of Dermatology* (9th ed.). Chichester: Wiley- Blackwell.

MedicineNet (2019). Group A streptococcal infections. Available at: https://www.medicinenet.com/script/main/art.asp?articlekey=143954 [Accessed: 28th November 2019].

MedlinePlus (2018). Bacterial infections. Available at: https://medlineplus.gov/bacterialinfections.html [Accessed: 24 July 2019].

MedlinePlus (2019). Aging changes in skin. Available at: https://medlineplus.gov/ency/article/004014.htm. [Accessed: 28 November 2019].

Melanoma Research Alliance (2019). Prevention. Available at: https://www.curemelanoma.org/about-melanoma/prevention/ [Accessed: 28 March 2019].

Mescher AL (2016). *Junqueira's Basic Histology*. New York: McGraw-Hill Education.

Mitchell E (2015). Gram-positive vs Gram-negative bacteria and the fight against HAIs. Available at: https://www.mayoclinic.org/diseasesconditions/staph-infections/symptomscauses/syc-20356221 [Accessed: 24 July 2019].

Morgan N (2014). What you need to know about transparent film dressings. *Wound Care Advisor*, 3(4). Available at: https://woundcareadvisor.com/what-you-need-to-know-about-transparent-film-dressings-vol3-no4/ [Accessed: 10 December 2019].

Mosby (2016). *Mosby's Medical Dictionary* (10th ed.) Philadelphia: Elsevier

National Eczema Association (2019a). Understanding your child's ezcema. Available at: https://nationaleczema.org/eczema/children/ [Accessed: 11 December 2019].

National Eczema Association (2019b). An Overview of the different types of eczema Available at: https://nationaleczema.org/eczema/types-of-eczema/. [Accessed: 11 December 2019].

National Eczema Society (2019). Topical steroids. Available at: http://www.eczema.org/corticosteroids [Accessed: 27 August 2019].

NCRAS (2012). Mortality, Incidence and Gender – malignant melanoma. *National Cancer Registration and Analysis Service*. Available at:http://www.ncin.org.uk/publications/data_briefings/mortality_incidence_and_gender_malignant_melanoma [Accessed: 28 March 2019].

Newson L (2015). Epidermoid and pilar cysts. *Patient*. Available: https://patient.info/doctor/epidermoid-and-pilar-cysts-sebaceous-cysts-pro [Accessed: 28 November 2019].

Newson L (2016). Viral rashes. *Patient*. Available at: https://patient.info/skin-conditions/viral-rashes [Accessed: 14 January 2020].

NHS (2016). Topical corticosteroids. Available at: https://www.nhs.uk/conditions/topical-steroids/ [Accessed: 24 July 2019].

NHS (2017a). Emollients. Available at: https://www.nhs.uk/conditions/emollients/ [Accessed: 27 August 2019].

NHS (2017b). Overview: Skin cancer (melanoma). Available at: https://www.nhs.uk/conditions/melanoma-skin-cancer/ [Accessed: 28 March 2019].

NHS (2017c). Balanitis. Available at: https://www.nhs.uk/conditions/balanitis/ [Accessed: 12 December 2019].

NHS (2017d). Chickenpox. Available at: https://www.nhs.uk/conditions/chickenpox/ [Accessed: 12 December 2019].

NHS (2017e). Cold sores. Available at: https://www.nhs.uk/conditions/cold-sore/ [Accessed: 28 March 2019].

NHS (2017f). Lichen planus. Available at: https://www.nhs.uk/conditions/lichen-planus/ [Accessed: 28 March 2019].

NHS (2017g). Molluscum contagiosum. Available at: https://www.nhs.uk/conditions/molluscum-contagiosum/ [Accessed: 28 March 2019].

NHS (2018a). Staph infection. Available at: https://www.nhs.uk/conditions/staphylococcal-infections/ [Accessed: 28 March 2019].

NHS (2018b). How do I clean a wound? Available at: https://www.nhs.uk/common-health-questions/accidents-first-aid-and-treatments/how-do-i-clean-a-wound/ [Accessed: 12 December 2019].

NHS (2018c). Nail problems. Available at: https://www.nhs.uk/conditions/nail-problems/ [Accessed: 28 March 2019].

NHS (2018d). Psoriasis. Available at: https://www.nhs.uk/conditions/psoriasis/ [Accessed: 11 December 2019].

NHS (2018e). Breastfeeding and thrush. Available at: https://www.nhs.uk/conditions/pregnancy-and-baby/breastfeeding-and-thrush/ [Accessed: 11 December 2019].

NHS (2018f). Head lice and nits. Available at: https://www.nhs.uk/conditions/head-lice-and-nits/ [Accessed: 12 December 2019].

NHS (2018g). Heat rash (prickly heat). Available at: https://www.nhs.uk/conditions/heat-rash-prickly-heat/ [Accessed: 11 December 2019].

NHS (2018h). Shingles. Available at: https://www.nhs.uk/conditions/shingles/ [Accessed: 28 March 2019].

NHS (2019a). Keloid scars. Available at: https://www.nhs.uk/live-well/healthy-body/keloid-scars/ [Accessed: 24 July 2019].

NHS (2019b). Treatment: Acne. Available at: https://www.nhs.uk/conditions/acne/treatment/ [Accessed: 12 December 2019].

NHS (2019d). Overview: Atopic eczema. Available at: https://www.nhs.uk/conditions/atopic-eczema/ [Accessed: 25 July 2019].

NHS (2019c). Vasculitis. Available at: https://www.nhs.uk/conditions/vasculitis/ [Accessed: 28 March 2019].

NHS Direct Wales (2019). Streptococcal infections. Available at: https://www.nhsdirect.wales.nhs.uk/ Encyclopaedia/s/article/streptococcalinfections/ [Accessed: 28th November 2019].

NHS Foundation Trust (2019). Henoch Schönlein Purpura (HSP). *NHS Great Ormond Street Hospital for Children*. Available at: https://www.gosh.nhs.uk/conditions-and-treatments/conditions-we-treat/henoch-sch-nlein-purpura-hsp [Accessed: 11 December 2019].

NHS Inform (2019a). Antibiotics. Available at: https://www.nhsinform.scot/tests-and-treatments/medicines-and-medical-aids/types-of-medicine/antibiotics [Accessed: 24 July 2019].

NHS Inform (2019b). Hand, foot and mouth disease. Available at: https://www.nhsinform.scot/illnesses-and-conditions/infections-and-poisoning/hand-foot-and-mouth-disease [Accessed: 11 December 2019].

NHS Inform (2019c). Chickenpox. Available at: https://www.nhsinform.scot/illnesses-and-conditions/infections-and-poisoning/chickenpox [Accessed: 12 December 2019].

NHS Inform (2019d). Shingles. Available at: https://www.nhsinform.scot/illnesses-and-conditions/infections-and-poisoning/shingles [Accessed: 12 December 2019].

NICE (2014). Warts and veruccae. Available at: https://cks.nice.org.uk/warts-and-verrucae#!topicSummary [Accessed: 14 January 2020].

NICE (2015) Pityriasis versicolor. Available at: https://cks.nice.org.uk/pityriasis-versicolor#toc [Accessed: 12 December 2019].

NICE (2016a). Pityriasis rosea. Available at: https://cks.nice.org.uk/pityriasis-rosea#!backgroundSub: [Accessed: 12 December 2019].

NICE (2016b). Sunlight exposure: risks and benefits overview. Available at: https://www.nice.org.uk/guidance/ng34 [Accessed: 28 March 2019].

NICE (2016c). Head lice. Available at: https://cks.nice.org.uk/head-lice#!scenario [Accessed: 12 December 2019].

NICE (2016d). Herpes simplex – oral. Available at: https://cks.nice.org.uk/herpes-simplex-oral#!prescribingInfoSub:2 [Accessed: 12 December 2019].

NICE (2016e). Insect bites and stings. Available at: https://cks.nice.org.uk/insect-bites-and-stings. [Accessed: 14 January 2020].

NICE (2017a). Paronychia - acute. Available at: https://cks.nice.org.uk/paronychia-acute#!topicSummary [Accessed: 14 January 2020].

NICE (2017b). Burns and scalds. Available at: https://cks.nice.org.uk/burns-and-scalds#!topicSummary [Accessed: 24 July 2019].

NICE (2017c). Candida – skin. Available at: https://cks.nice.org.uk/candida-skin#!topicSummary [Accessed: 12 December 2019].

NICE (2017d). Candida – oral. Available at: https://cks.nice.org.uk/candida-oral#!management [Accessed: 12 December 2019].

NICE (2017e). Candida – female genital. Available at: https://cks.nice.org.uk/candida-female-genital#toc [Accessed: 12 December 2019].

NICE (2017f). Melanoma and pigmented lesions. Available at: https://cks.nice.org.uk/melanoma-and-pigmented-lesions#!diagnosis [Accessed: 28 March 2019].

NICE (2017g). Boils, carbuncles and staphylococcal carriage. Available at: https://cks.nice.org.uk/boils-carbuncles-and-staphylococcal-carriage#toc [Accessed: 12 December 2019].

NICE (2017h). Parvovirus B19 infection. Available at: https://cks.nice.org.uk/parvovirus-b19-infection#!topicSummary [Accessed: 12 December 2019].

NICE (2018a) Dermatitis – contact. Available at: https://cks.nice.org.uk/dermatitis-contact#!scenario [Accessed: 12 December 2019].

NICE (2018b). Eczema – atopic. Available at: https://cks.nice.org.uk/eczema-atopic [Accessed: 28 March 2019].

NICE (2018c). Psoriasis. Available at: https://cks.nice.org.uk/psoriasis [Accessed: 28 March 2019].

NICE (2018d). Fungal nail infection. Available at: https://cks.nice.org.uk/fungal-nail-infection [Accessed: 27 July 2019].

NICE (2018e). Fungal skin infection body and groin. Available at: https://cks.nice.org.uk/fungal-skin-infection-body-and-groin#!scenario. [Accessed: 12 December 2019].

NICE (2018f). Balanitis. Available at: https://cks.nice.org.uk/balanitis#!topicSummary. [Accessed: 12 December 2019].

NICE (2018g). Nappy Rash. Available at: https://cks.nice.org.uk/nappy-rash#toc [Accessed: 12 December 2019].

NICE (2018h). Otitis externa. Available at: https://cks.nice.org.uk/otitis-externa#!scenarioRecommendation:14 [Accessed: 12 December 2019].

NICE (2018i). Acne vulgaris: management of acne vulgaris in primary care. Available at: https://cks.nice.org.uk/acne-vulgaris#!scenarioRecommendation [Accessed: 28 March 2019].

NICE (2018j). Chickenpox. Available at: https://cks.nice.org.uk/chickenpox#!scenario [Accessed: 12 December 2019].

NICE (2018k). Impetigo. Available at: https://cks.nice.org.uk/impetigo#!topicSummary [Accessed: 14 January 2020].

NICE (2018l). Rosacea acne. Available at: https://cks.nice.org.uk/rosacea-acne#!topicSummary [Accessed: 14 January 2020].

NICE (2018m). Scarlet fever. Available at: https://cks.nice.org.uk/scarlet-fever#!topicSummary [Accessed: 14 January 2020].

NICE (2018n). Urticaria. Available at: https://cks.nice.org.uk/urticaria#!topicSummary [Accessed: 14 January 2020].

NICE (2019a). Summary of antimicrobial prescribing guidance – managing common infections. Available at: https://www.nice.org.uk/about/what-we-do/our-programmes/nice-guidance/antimicrobial-prescribing-guidelines [Accessed: 20 April 2019].

NICE (2019b). Clinical Knowledge Summaries. Available at: https://cks.nice.org.uk/#?char=A [Accessed: 24 July 2019].

NICE (2019c). Emollient creams and ointments, paraffin-containing. Available at: https://bnf.nice.org.uk/medicinal-forms/emollient-creams-and-ointments-paraffin-containing.html [Accessed 27: August 2019].

NICE (2019d). Corticosteroids – topical (skin), nose, and eyes. Available at: https://cks.nice.org.uk/corticosteroids-topical-skin-nose-and-eyes [Accessed: 28 March 2019].

NICE (2019e). Fludroxycortide. Available at: https://bnf.nice.org.uk/drug/fludroxycortide.html [Accessed: 12 December 2019].

NICE (2019f). Seborrhoeic dermatitis. Available at: https://cks.nice.org.uk/seborrhoeic-dermatitis#!topicSummary. [Accessed: 11 December 2019].

NICE (2019g). Suspected cancer recognition and referral. Available at: https://www.nice.org.uk/guidance/ng12 [Accessed: 28 March 2019].

NICE (2019h). Cellulitis – acute. Available at: https://cks.nice.org.uk/cellulitis-acute#!prescribingInfo [Accessed: 12 December 2019].

NICE (2019i). Shingles. Available at: https://cks.nice.org.uk/shingles#!prescribingInfo [Accessed: 12 December 2019].

NICE (2019j). Fever in under 5s: assessment and initial management. Available at: https://www.nice. org.uk/guidance/ng143 [Accessed: 8 January 2020].

Oakley A (2015). Melanoma. Available at: https://www.dermnetnz.org/topics/melanoma/. *DermNet NZ*. [Accessed: 10 May 2019].

ONS (2003). SunSmart protection survey. *Office of National Statistics*. London: Cancer Research UK. Online Clinic (2019). *Haelan Tape*. Available at: https://www.theonlineclinic.co.uk/ haelan-tape.asp. [Accessed: 11 December 2019].

Onselen JV (2016). Skin assessment and language of dermatology. *Nursing in Practice*. Available at: https://tinyurl.com/yd59c884 [Accessed: 11 December 2018].

Oskeritzian CA (2012). Mast cells and wound healing, *Advances in Wound Care*. 1(1): 23–28.

Ovaere P, Lippens S, Vandenabeele P and Declercq W (2009). The emerging roles of serine protease cascades in the epidermis. *Trends in Biochemical Sciences*, 34(9): 453–463.

Pavelka M and Roth J (2010). *Functional Ultrastructure*. Vienna: Springer.

PCDS (2016a). Eczema: discoid (syn. Nummular) eczema. *Primary Care Dermatology Society*. Available at: http://www.pcds.org.uk/clinical-guidance/eczema-discoid-syn.-nummular-eczema [Accessed: 28 March 2019].

PCDS (2016b). Candidal infection (syn. candidiasis; candidiosis; moniliasis). *Primary Care Dermatology Society*. Available at: http://www.pcds.org.uk/clinical-guidance/candida-infection [Accessed: 11 December 2019].

PCDS (2016c). Intertrigo. *Primary Care Dermatology Society*. Available at: http://www.pcds.org.uk/ clinical-guidance/intertrigo#management [Accessed: 11 December 2019].

PCDS (2017a). Tinea corporis (body), cruris (groin) and incogto (steroid exacerbated). *Primary Care Dermatology Society*. Available at: http://www.pcds.org.uk/clinical-guidance/tinea-corporis-body-cruris-groin-and-incognito-steroid-exacerbated#management. [Accessed: 12 December 2019].

PCDS (2017b). Melanoma: lentigo maligna melanoma (including lentigo maligna) *Primary Care Dermatology Society*. Available at: http://www.pcds.org.uk/clinical-guidance/lentigo-maligna-melanoma-and-lentigo-maligna [Accessed: 28 March 2019].

PCDS (2018a). Folliculitis and boils. *Primary Care Dermatology Society*. Available at: http://www. pcds.org.uk/clinical-guidance/folliculitis-an-overview#management [Accessed: 12 December 2019].

PCDS (2018b). Rosacea. *Primary Care Dermatology Society*. Available at: http://www.pcds.org.uk/ clinical-guidance/rosacea [Accessed: 28 March 2019].

PCDS (2018c). Lichen planus. Available at: http://www.pcds.org.uk/clinical-guidance/lichen-planus#management. [Accessed: 14 January 2020].

PCDS (2019a). Eczema: hand (and foot) eczema. *Primary Care Dermatology Society*. Available at: http://www.pcds.org.uk/clinical-guidance/eczema-hand-dermatitis#management [Accessed: 12 December 2019].

PCDS (2019b). Tinea capitis (scalp). *Primary Care Dermatology Society*. Available at: http://www. pcds.org.uk/clinical-guidance/tinea-capitis-scalp#management [Accessed: 12 December 2019].

PCDS (2019c). Acne: acne vulgaris. *Primary Care Dermatology Society*. Available at: http://www. pcds.org.uk/clinical-guidance/acne-vulgaris [Accessed: 27 August 2019].

PCDS (2019d). Vasculitis. *Primary Care Dermatology Society*. Available at: http://www.pcds.org.uk/ clinical-guidance/vasculitis-and-capillaritis#management [Accessed: 11 December 2019].

PCDS (2019e). lichen planus – folicular Lichen planus. *Primary Care Dermatology Society*. Available at: http://www.pcds.org.uk/clinical-guidance/lichen-planus-follicular-lichen-planus [Accessed: 12 December 2019].

Public Health England (2018a). Antibiotic awareness: posters and leaflets. Available at: https://www.gov.uk/government/publications/european-antibiotic-awareness-day-and-antibiotic-guardian-posters-and-leaflets [Accessed: 28 March 2019].

Public Health England (2018b). Tick bite marks and prevention of Lyme disease: resources. Available at: https://www.gov.uk/government/publications/tick-bite-risks-and-prevention-of-lyme-disease [Accessed: 28 March 2019].

Public Health England (2019). Managing common infections: guidance for primary care. Available at: https://www.gov.uk/government/publications/managing-common-infections-guidance-for-primary-care [Accessed: 29 March 2019].

Rollins (2004). Comparative characteristics of Gram-positive and Gram-negative bacteria. Available at: https://science.umd.edu/classroom/bsci424/BSCI223WebSiteFiles/GramPosvsGramNeg.htm [Accessed: 6 August 2019].

Salama A (2016). IgA Vasculitis (Henoch-Schönlein-Purpura). Available at: https://www.vasculitis.org.uk/about-vasculitis/henoch-schonlein-purpura [Accessed: 28 March 2019].

Sandeen D (2019). How often should I shampoo black hair? Available at: https://www.liveabout.com/how-often-should-i-shampoo-black-hair-400058 [Accessed: 23 January 2020].

Skin Authority (2019). Skin Explained. Available at: http://www.skinauthority.com/Skin-Explained [Accessed: 20 November 2019].

Smith Y (2019). What is subcutaneous tissue? Available at: https://www.news-medical.net/health/What-is-Subcutaneous-Tissue.aspx. [Accessed: 20 November 2019].

Sommers M (2011). Color awareness: A must for patient assessment. Available at: https://www.americannursetoday.com/color-awareness-a-must-for-patient-assessment/ [Accessed: 28 November 2019].

Stanway A (2015). Staphylococcal skin infection. *DermNetNZ*. Available: https://dermnetnz.org/topics/staphylococcal-skin-infection/. [Accessed: 28 November 2019].

Starr O (2017). Scabies. Available at: https://patient.info/skin-conditions/skin rashes/scabies [Accessed: 28 March 2019].

Starr O (2018). Athlete's Foot: Tinea Pedis. *Patient*. Available at: https://patient.info/infections/fungal-infections/athletes-foot-tinea-pedis [Accessed: August 2019].

Tortora GJ and Derrickson BH (2017). *Principles of Anatomy and Physiology* (15th ed.). Hoboken: John Wiley Inc.

Tsatmali M, Ancans J and Thody AJ (2002). Melanocyte function and its control by melanocortin peptides. *Journal of Histochemistry & Cytochemistry*, 50(2): 125–133.

THT (2019). Herpes. *Terence Higgins Trust*. Available at: https://www.tht.org.uk/hiv-and-sexual-health/sexual-health/stis/herpes [Accessed: 12 December 2019].

Tucker R (2011). What evidence is there for moisturisers? *Pharmaceutical Journal Online*. Available at: https://www.pharmaceutical-journal.com/cpd-and-learning/learning-article/what-evidence-is-there-for-moisturisers/11073483.article?firstPass=false [Accessed: 28 March 2019].

Van Zuuren EJ et al. (2017). Emollients and moisturisers for eczema. *Cochrane*. Available at: https://www.cochrane.org/CD012119/SKIN_emollients-andmoisturisers-eczema [Accessed: 28 March 2019].

Walker FM et al. (2013). Using the 7-point checklist as a diagnostic aid for pigmented skin lesions in general practice: a diagnostic validation study. *British Journal of General Practice*, 63(610): 345–353.

Walter SD, King WD and Marrett LD (1999). Association of cutaneous malignant melanoma with intermittent exposure to ultraviolet radiation: results of a case–control study in Ontario, Canada. *International Journal of Epidemiology*, 28: 418–427.

WebMD (2018). Bacteria and Viral infections. Available at: https://www.webmd.com/a-to-z- guides/ bacterial-and-viral-infections#1 [Accessed: 24 July 2019].

Woo M (2019). Why don't newborns have tears or sweat? *LiveScience*. Available at: https://www. livescience.com/newborns-no-tears-or-sweat.html [Accessed: 28 November 2019].

Williams HC, Dellavalle RP and Garner S (2012). Acne vulgaris. *Lancet*, 379(9813): 361–72.

World Health Organization (2018). Antibiotic resistance. Available at: https://www.who.int/news-room/fact-sheets/detail/antibiotic-resistance [Accessed: 24 July 2019].

Wounds International (2013). Soft silicone dressing made easy. Available at: https://www. woundsinternational.com/download/resource/6106. [Accessed: 10 December 2019].

Young B, O'Dowd G and Woodford P (2013). *Wheater's Functional Histology* (6th ed.). Philadelphia: Churchill Livingstone.

Index

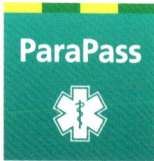

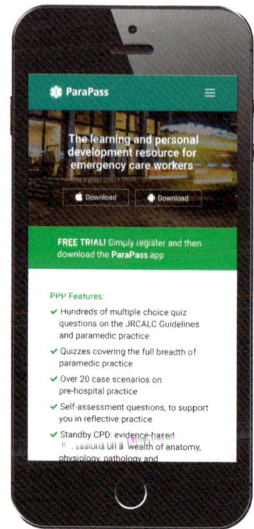

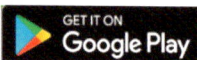

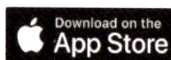

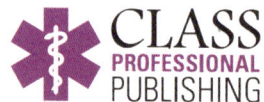